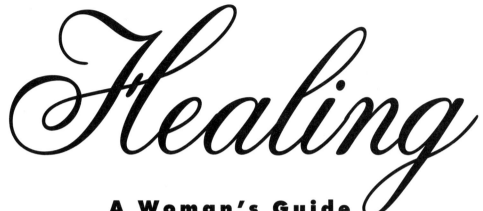

Healing

A Woman's Guide
To Lumpectomy and
Radiation Therapy

*R*osalind D. Benedet, N.P., M.S.N.

and

*M*ark C. Rounsaville, M.D.

Benedet Publishing
San Francisco

The recommendations are not intended to replace or conflict with the advice given to you by your doctors and other health-care professionals, and we recommend that you follow their advice.

Library of Congress Catalog Card Number 95-96248
ISBN 0-9637917-1-0

Illustrations by Shannon Abbey
Edited by Edith A. Folb, Ph.D.
Production Coordination by M.J. Coleman
Cover Design by Curium Design
Typesetting by Bonnie Monohan

Benedet Publishing
220 Montgomery Street
Penthouse No. 2
San Francisco, California 94104

*This book is dedicated
in memory of*
Judy Diane Hill
1947–1991

*Those whom we have loved
are with us always, for love never dies.*

—With Fond Remembrances,
Flavia Weedn, 1988

Thanks

The thoughts and efforts of many people have gone into this book. We sincerely appreciate each person's contribution.

Shannon Abbey

Mellownee Bassett

Derrick Bowyer

Pattie Bryson

Elizabeth Burrell

Richard Cohen, M.D.

M.J. Coleman

Erika P. Donald

Edith Folb

Jane Horii

Sharron Long

Linda T. Miller, P.T.

Bonnie Monohan

Michael Small, M.D.

Evan Sornstein

Joy Sornstein

Theresa Thompson

Mary Wohlford

A special thank you to:

M.J. Coleman

Edith Folb

Sharron Long

Table of Contents

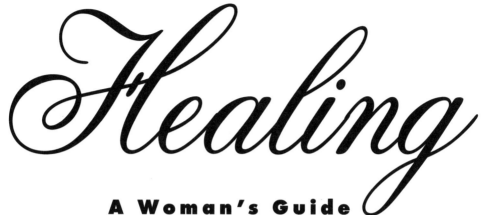

Healing

A Woman's Guide
To Lumpectomy and
Radiation Therapy

About This Guide

This guide is designed to aid your physical and emotional healing. It offers practical and easy-to-understand information about your *lumpectomy* and *radiation therapy*. It also lets you know what to do on a day-to-day basis. Other treatments, such as chemotherapy and hormonal therapy, are briefly covered. Knowing what to expect and how to take care of yourself should lessen many of your concerns and allow you to actively participate in your treatment plan and recovery.

Though you will have the support and care of a team of health professionals, you are truly the most important person on that team. A strong desire and determination to heal, faith and humor, open patient-doctor relationships, and realistic information about what lies ahead will give you the tools you need to speed your recovery.

Your doctors and nurses are your best sources of information. The information in this guide will add to their advice.

We hope this guide will contribute to your recovery and healing.

1.

Before Your Surgery

Talking with Your Doctors

*I*n the weeks and months to come, you'll probably have a number of questions and concerns about your treatment and healing process. You are encouraged to bring all your questions and concerns to your doctors. The unknown can be very scary, but information about what lies ahead can reduce some of the anxiety that you may feel. Being informed about your treatment plan also allows you to play an active role in your recovery.

It's very important to develop an open relationship with your doctors. This depends on how frankly you are able to speak with your doctors. They need to know what you're thinking and feeling so that they can prescribe the best treatment and resources for you. They also need to know how much or how little information you want from them.

Write down your questions and concerns as you think of them and bring that list with you to your visits. Remember, there is no such thing as a "silly" or "dumb" question.

It is sometimes difficult to remember discussions with your doctors. You may find it helpful to take notes and/or ask a friend along to help you remember what is said. Also, you can ask your doctor if you may tape-record your conversation.

Don't be shy about asking the same questions over again. It's not always easy to take in all that the doctor is saying. Simple statements like, "I know that I asked this before, but I couldn't remember all that you said" or "Can we talk about it again?" help both you and your doctor to focus on important information.

Ask your doctors about the best method for talking to them about your concerns: By telephone? At a special appointment? At a regular visit, with more time scheduled in for discussion?

Remember, you are the best judge of your own body — don't ever be embarrassed to bring your concerns to the attention of your health care providers.

A Brief Overview of Your Treatment

Lumpectomy with radiation therapy is an important advancement in the treatment of breast cancer, because it allows your doctors to effectively treat breast cancer locally (in the breast and chest area) while preserving your breast. While many women are relieved that they will keep their breast, some women worry that a lumpectomy may not be as "safe" as a mastectomy.

It's important to know that the combination of lumpectomy with radiation therapy is just as effective as mastectomy. This has been proven in many research studies in the United States and Europe. This research is so well accepted that in June 1990 the National Institute of Health (NIH) Consensus Conference concluded that lumpectomy with radiation therapy is *preferable* to mastectomy for Stage I and Stage II breast cancer because it provides the same survival rate and preserves the breast. So the combination of lumpectomy followed by radiation therapy is a safe, strong, and effective treatment for breast cancer.

Lumpectomy — A Breast Conservation Treatment

Lumpectomy is a surgical procedure that removes the cancer and a rim of healthy tissue around the tumor. It is called a *breast conservation procedure*. This means that the appearance of your breast should not be dramatically changed.

This procedure may be done in a number of ways. You may be given either a local or a general anesthesia. If the initial biopsy removed your tumor, that biopsy could serve as the lumpectomy. However, if a significant amount of the tumor is left in the breast, after your initial biopsy, your surgeon and your radiation doctor may recommend that more tissue be removed. This additional surgery may be called a *re-excision*, a *lumpectomy*, a *segmental mastectomy*, a *partial mastectomy*, or a *tylectomy*. These words are sometimes used interchangeably.

The actual words that are used do not matter. What is important is that you know how much tissue will be removed and how your breast will look after the surgery. Though your breast may be smaller, it should retain its original shape. If you are concerned with the appearance of your breast after surgery, you may want to seek a second opinion.

Lymph Node Surgery

Commonly, some of the lymph nodes in the armpit region of the affected breast are surgically removed to determine if the cancer has spread. This surgery is called an *axillary node sampling* or a *dissection*. It's usually done at the time of the re-excision, or if a re-excision is not needed, in a separate operation for that purpose. General anesthesia is given for this procedure. Usually, a separate incision from the lumpectomy is made in the underarm region. By making two separate incisions, one incision for the lumpectomy and another for the axillary surgery, the surgeon is usually able to keep both incisions small.

Removing the lymph nodes, as with any surgical or medical procedure, contains both benefits and risks. The main benefit is to obtain information about the likelihood that cancer cells have left the breast. This helps determine whether chemotherapy and/or hormonal therapy (i.e., tamoxifen) is needed. One potential risk is that sometimes a sensory nerve (a nerve responsible for sensation or feeling) is cut. This may result in temporary or permanent numbness in the affected armpit and under-arm area. Another risk is a condition called *lymphedema*. Lymphedema is a chronic swelling of the hand and/or arm on the side of the axillary lymph node surgery. There is more information about lymphedema in Chapter 3. If you are concerned about these issues, talk with your surgeon about whether your lymph nodes need to be removed or whether this is an optional procedure, in your case.

Radiation Therapy

In a few weeks following your surgery, after you have healed, you will begin your radiation therapy. Radiation therapy is provided during out-patient visits to the radiation treatment center, Monday through Friday, for about five weeks to eight weeks. Radiation therapy is generally well tolerated and most women continue to enjoy an active life during therapy. Sometimes, chemotherapy is given before or after radiation therapy.

Informed Consent

Before surgery and radiation therapy, you will be asked to read and sign consent forms. Signing the forms means that you have been told about the procedures and their potential risks. It also means that you understand your options and agree to have the recommended procedures performed.

You should be given the forms in advance of your treatment so that you can look them over and raise any questions or concerns with your surgeon. Here are some of the questions you might want to ask:

LUMPECTOMY QUESTIONS

◆ What kind of procedure are you recommending?

◆ How much tissue will be removed?

◆ Where will the incision be located and how large will it be?

◆ What will my breast look like after the lumpectomy?

◆ What are the risks and side effects of a lumpectomy?

◆ What type of anesthesia will I have? Local? General?

◆ How long will I be in the hospital? Same day discharge? Overnight?

AXILLARY NODE SURGERY QUESTIONS

◆ Are the lymph nodes in my armpit going to be removed?

◆ About how many lymph nodes will be removed?

◆ Where will the incision be located and how large will it be?

◆ What will my underarm area look like after the axillary node sampling/dissection?

◆ What are the risks and side effects of an axillary node sampling?

◆ How long will I be in the hospital? Same day discharge? Overnight?

A Second Opinion

Sometimes, even after several discussions with your doctors, you may still feel unclear and uncertain about the treatment plan. Is it right for you? If you have questions or doubts, seek a second opinion. Having the opportunity to discuss your concerns and options with different cancer specialists may clear up lingering questions. Your doctors will not feel "offended" if you seek a second opinion. Quite the contrary. Your doctors want you to fully understand the procedures they have recommended, and they sincerely want you to feel that you are making the best personal choice. Being an active member in your treatment plan helps you develop and maintain a positive attitude which can only enhance your recovery.

2.

Your Hospital Stay

Preparing for Surgery

*H*ospital procedures differ. But, most likely, you'll be asked to have routine tests, such as blood tests and a chest x-ray, done one or two days before your surgery. You'll probably be admitted to the hospital the morning of your surgery and discharged later on the same day or the next morning.

We suggest you pack lightly since your stay in the hospital will be a short one. Most hospitals will provide for your personal needs (i.e., toothpaste, soap, body lotion). If you prefer, bring your own favorite grooming products (i.e., face cream, hand lotion, and so on). Since all of your jewelry, including rings and earrings, will be removed before surgery, you may decide to leave these at home.

When packing, think about bringing along some special clothing that will make it easier for you to dress after surgery. Here are some suggested items:

◆ A loose-fitting blouse, shirt, or dress that buttons in the front. It will be easier for you to put on than a pull-on garment or one that buttons or zips in the back.

◆ A soft tee shirt or camisole. This will be much more comfortable than a bra after your surgery.

Before Your Surgery

When it's time for your surgery, you'll be asked to undress completely and put on a hospital gown. Your jewelry, wallet, and other personal items will be taken and placed in a secure place; these will be returned to you after surgery. If you wear dentures, a hearing aid, contact lenses, or glasses, they, too, will be safely put away and brought to your hospital room after your surgery. Just before your surgery, you may be given some medication to help you relax.

Having General Anesthesia

You'll be taken to the operating room on a gurney (a bed with wheels) or in a wheelchair; or you may be asked to walk, accompanied by a nurse. Before you fall asleep, an intravenous line (IV) will be put into your arm to provide you with necessary medications and fluids. The surgery itself will take about two hours.

After Your Surgery

When you wake up in the operating room, one of the first sensations you may notice is that you are cold. You will be covered with a warm blanket. From the operating room, you'll be brought to the recovery room. In the recovery room, a nurse will frequently check your temperature, pulse, blood pressure, and your dressing. The nurse will also make sure you are comfortable and will give you medication for pain or nausea, if needed.

You will spend about an hour in the recovery room before being brought to your own hospital room and settled into your bed. Your nurse will check in on you frequently. If you feel pain or nausea, you'll be given medication.

Although visitors are not allowed in the recovery room, you may have people come to see you as soon as you are settled in your own hospital room.

Preparing for Discharge from the Hospital

When you're fully awake, usually a couple of hours after being returned to your hospital room, you'll be encouraged to sit up in bed, take deep breaths, and cough. This helps clear out your lungs and prevents any potential lung complications.

You'll be given clear liquids, such as Jell-O, clear broth, and tea, four to six hours after surgery. Your IV will be removed as soon as you begin drinking liquids and as long as your temperature is normal and no medications need to be given by IV. About four to six hours after your surgery, you'll be asked to get up from your bed and walk. Your nurse will help you.

By evening, most women are ready and eager to go home. Before you're released from the hospital, your nurse will prepare you for discharge. She will carefully explain the following:

1. How to care for yourself at home.

2. How to take your pain medication. She'll give you your prescription at that time.

3. When your surgeon wants to see you for a follow-up visit (usually about five days after surgery).

4. How to take care of your drain, if you have a drain. See page 21 for detailed drain-care instructions.

3.

Your Recovery at Home

Many women say they feel surprisingly well the second day after surgery. The physical discomfort from a lumpectomy is generally minimal; it usually feels like the discomfort that is felt after a breast biopsy. However, your armpit, where the lymph nodes have been removed, will probably be sore.

Depending on where the incision is located on your breast, you may find that wearing a bra during the day and at night is more comfortable than going without one. Since your breast may be swollen, make sure that the cup is not too tight. Generally, the most comfortable bra is one that has a soft unlined cup without an underwire. On the other hand, you may find that a soft tee shirt or camisole is more comfortable. Clothes that button in the front are usually the most comfortable to wear during the first few days after surgery.

If you experience pain or discomfort, take your prescribed medication as needed. Many women resist taking pain medication because they worry about becoming dependent on it. Remember that pain medication is generally needed only for a few days and nights, so dependency is not really an issue. Sometimes an over-the-counter pain medication can be as effective as a prescribed one. Ask your doctor to suggest one. Do not take medication that contains aspirin. Aspirin prolongs bleeding time and should be avoided one week before and after surgery. In the long run, if you take pain medication regularly, as directed, rather than taking it when the pain gets to be "too much," you'll be more comfortable and will need less medication. Being comfortable allows you to be physically active and to get your needed rest. Both are important for healing and recovery.

You may notice that you have less energy than you normally do. Don't be discouraged; slowly, your energy will increase. You may also notice that your upper arm, armpit, and breast are temporarily swollen from the surgery. To help reduce swelling, place your arm comfortably on several pillows so that your arm is resting at a level higher than your heart. In addition, perform the "Arm Pumps" exercise demonstrated on page 38 about three times a day.

Bed rest is not encouraged, because inactivity and bed rest tend to lead to more fatigue. We recommend that you stay physically active. However, some women do benefit from a nap during the day. A good rule of thumb is to do what you feel capable of doing.

A FEW GUIDELINES FOR APPROPRIATE LEVELS OF ACTIVITY:

◆ Use your affected arm. Gentle motions are recommended. Try not to hold your arm stiffly against your body. Make a special effort to relax your neck, shoulder, and arm on your affected side. (See Chapter 5 for more information on arm exercises.)

◆ Allow family and friends to help you with housework and the preparation of meals. If you want, you may do some moderate housework such as preparing a simple meal or washing a few dishes. Avoid strenuous lifting, pushing, or pulling, particularly with your affected arm.

Looking at Your Breast

Although you may feel relieved that you have kept your breast, you may also feel sad and disappointed over the change in the appearance of your breast. A scar on any part of your body can be upsetting, and it is common and normal to be particularly concerned with a scar on your breast. It should be comforting to know that, in time, scars fade and slight depressions fill in.

The first time you look at your breast in the mirror can be a difficult moment. Some women want to look at their breast right away, immediately after surgery; others put off looking for a few weeks. There is no right way or right time. You'll know when you are ready. Looking at your breast is important to make sure your incisions are healing properly and to get comfortable with the changes in your body.

You may notice bruising and swelling in the affected breast, armpit, and the underarm area. The bruising and swelling are temporary and will slowly disappear. Sometimes, a pocket of fluid develops in the armpit. This is called a *seroma*. If you develop a seroma, let your surgeon know. When you bring your arm against your body, the seroma can feel uncomfortably large. A seroma always feels much larger than it actually is. It usually goes away by itself in a few weeks. However, you and your surgeon may decide that you will be more comfortable if it's drained. Draining a seroma is done in your doctor's office. A very small needle is inserted into the seroma, and the fluid is removed. It's a quick and relatively painless procedure.

Caring for Your Incisions

Although taking care of your incisions may sound intimidating, it is really a straightforward and easily managed process. Remember, you may have two incisions, one on your breast and the other in the under-arm area where some of your lymph nodes were removed. When you are discharged, you may have a small dressing over your incisions. If so, just keep the dressing dry. The incisions won't heal properly if the dressing stays wet. Your surgeon will either ask you to remove the dressing in one or two days, or the dressing will be removed at your follow-up visit, about five days after your surgery. Sometimes the dressing is removed before you go home from the hospital.

Your incisions may be closed with regular stitches that need to be removed by your surgeon at your first follow-up visit. Or, your incisions may be closed with absorbable stitches that "disappear" on their own. Absorbable stitches are covered with steri-strips (a special type of tape). The steri-strips will fall off by themselves, about 10 days after surgery. If the steri-strips get wet, just pat them dry.

Although an infection at the site of the incisions is unlikely, you should observe the incisions for signs of increased redness, drainage, swelling, warmth, or pain. If any of these conditions develop, call your surgeon.

Taking Care of Your Drain

*A*bout half of the women who have an axillary node sampling have a drain placed in the underarm area. If you don't have a drain, you can skip this section. If you're not sure whether you have one or not, ask your surgeon or hospital nurse.

Drains may be inconvenient and are not very pretty to look at, but they serve a necessary function. They may be placed under the skin during surgery to remove blood and fluids that collect as part of the healing process. If you have a drain in your underarm area, it may be removed before you are discharged from the hospital. It is more likely, however, that you will go home with your drain in place.

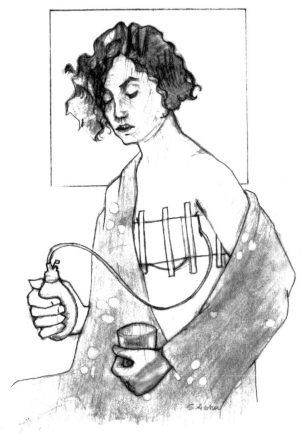

If you do go home with the drain in place, you will need to empty it.

Instructions for Emptying Your Drain

*E*mptying your own drain is easy. Your nurse will review the following instructions with you before your discharge from the hospital:

1. Wash your hands.

2. Remove the plug from the pouring spout and pour the contents out.

3. Measure the contents. A measuring cup may be used.

4. Flatten the drainage container and replace the plug into the spout.

5. Record the date, time, and amount of drainage. (See page 108 for "Drain Care Chart.")

6. Empty the container two times a day (i.e., when you get up in the morning and before going to sleep at night).

7. Look at the skin around the drain. If you notice increased redness, swelling, warmth, pus, or pain, call your surgeon.

8. Safety-pin your drain to your blouse or underclothes.

9. Always keep your drain below the level of your armpit.

As you heal you will notice that you will have less drainage, and the color of the drainage will change from red to light pink, to a light, straw-colored yellow.

INSTRUCTIONS FOR CHANGING YOUR DRAIN DRESSING

You may have a drain dressing. If so, just keep the dressing dry. If the doctor wants you to change the dressing, you will change it just once a day, or whenever it gets wet. Your nurse will review the following steps with you before you are discharged from the hospital:

1. Wash your hands.

2. Remove the old dressing and throw it away.

3. Look at the skin around the drain. If you notice increased redness, swelling, warmth, pus, or pain, call your surgeon.

4. Place two four-inch-by-four-inch sterile gauze pads on top of each other. Cut a two-inch slit in each dressing with clean scissors.

5. Place the dressing on the skin, where the tube comes out of your body. Then place the drain tube within the slit.

6. Tape the dressing in place. Use paper first-aid tape if you are allergic to adhesive tape.

7. Wash your hands again.

8. Safety-pin your drain to your blouse or underclothes.

9. Always keep your drain below the level of your armpit.

Noting Sensory Changes

You are encouraged to touch your incisions and scar, affected breast, and underarm to discover the different sensations — or lack of sensations — you may experience. You won't hurt yourself by doing this. This way, you'll find out which areas have lost feeling or are extremely sensitive to touch. You'll also find out what does or does not feel good to the touch.

As your incisions heal, a scar will form. At first, the scar will be pink, but over time, about a year and a half, the scar should fade. When you run your finger over the scar, you may notice that it has a firm ridge. This ridge, called a healing ridge, is normal. In time, the ridge will soften. While the scar is healing, it may itch. Massaging vitamin E oil into the scar may soften the scar and make it feel more comfortable.

Over the course of the first year or so you may feel an occasional sharp pain, heaviness, and burning or dull aching in your affected breast, armpit, and arm. These normal sensations indicate that the nerve endings are growing back. These sensations may vary. They may increase with tiredness, emotional stress, or changes in the weather, but will lessen in about a year.

If lymph nodes have been removed from under your armpit, some of the nerves there may be cut or stretched. As a result, you may feel an area of numbness or decreased feeling in your armpit and on the back of that arm. You may regain some or most of the sensation there, over the course of the year.

As you can see, you will probably experience many different sensations in your affected breast, arm, and underarm areas. If you know what to expect, these sensations won't be cause for worry.

Preventing Lymphedema: Special Nail, Hand, and Arm Care

*A*fter lymph node surgery, there is no reason why you can't use your hand and arm in a normal way, and enjoy doing all the things you did before the surgery. However, you will need to give some *lifelong,* special attention to your nails, hand, and arm on the side of your surgery to prevent a possible complication called *lymphedema.* Lymphedema is a chronic swelling of the hand and/or arm.

In an axillary node sampling, the lymph nodes under the arm next to the affected breast are removed. The removal of these underarm lymph nodes can cause the lymphatic drainage system (primarily made up of lymph nodes, lymph vessels, and lymph fluid) in your affected hand and arm to become sluggish. Since this system is an important part of your overall immune system and helps keep infections in check, this sluggishness increases the risk of infection in the affected side. An injury or an untreated infection of your affected hand, arm, or underarm area may lead to lymphedema.

It is important to ask your doctor how many lymph nodes were removed during surgery to determine what your risk is of developing lymphedema. The greater the number of lymph nodes that have been removed, the greater the risk for developing lymphedema. Attempting to remove all the lymph nodes — a *lymph node dissection* — increases the risk.

Although lymphedema can and should be treated, it cannot be cured. Lymphedema may develop soon after surgery or many years later. If swelling does develop, it is important to start treatment as soon as possible. See page 116 for information on how to contact an expert in treating lymphedema.

The following *lifelong* guidelines will help you prevent lymphedema:

Stay physically active. If you haven't been physically active or haven't done physical exercises regularly, it is important to gradually build up your physical stamina. General physical activity, such as walking, is a good beginning. Physical activity causes the muscles throughout your body to contract, and this encourages lymphatic drainage. Building muscle strength in both arms is also desirable since good muscle tone is a safeguard against injuring your arm. Many times, a woman will injure her arm by carrying a seemingly light package or briefcase that turns out to be too heavy for her.

Protect your nails, hand, arm, and underarm on the affected side from injury. Injury can lead to an infection as well as chronic swelling. Give yourself gentle manicures; don't cut your cuticles and avoid artificial nails — they are a source of fungal infections. Bring your own manicuring tools to your manicurist if you have your nails done professionally. Wear protective gloves while performing jobs that might lead to injury, such as home maintenance, yard work, and baking. Wear long-sleeved clothes, insect repellent, and sunscreen to protect against sunburn and insect bites. Finally, use an electric razor if you shave under your arms.

If you injure your hand or arm, treat the injury appropriately. Vigorously wash the wound with soap and warm water several times a day. Apply antibiotic lotion to the wound each time you wash. Cover the wound with a bandage and keep the bandage dry. If the injury looks like it is getting infected (i.e., red, swelling, pus, or pain), see your doctor immediately for antibiotic therapy.

Lifelong Tips to Avoid Injuring Your Hand and Arm

◆ Avoid carrying heavy objects, such as handbags, briefcases, or suitcases, on the affected side.

◆ Avoid having blood drawn, injections, or chemotherapy in the affected arm.

◆ Avoid acupuncture in the affected arm.

◆ Avoid having blood pressure taken on the affected arm.

4.

Getting Back to Your Normal Routines

Bathing and Showering

You may take a bath as soon as you wish. However, if you have a dressing over your incision, do not get it wet. To make sure you don't get your dressing wet, you may need help while bathing; or you might choose to take a sponge bath. If you have a drain, don't submerge your chest under water.

After your drain and dressing have been removed by your surgeon, you're free to shower. At first, stand with your back to the showerhead to avoid the full force of the water on your incision. It's okay if your steri-strips get wet; just pat them dry with a towel. Don't be afraid to touch your incision. You will not hurt anything. Since the incision in your armpit may be numb, it may feel as if you're washing someone else.

Sleeping

It's all right to sleep in any position you find comfortable. Many women find that lying on their back, with pillows under their affected arm, is the most comfortable position. If you enjoy sleeping on your side, lie on your unaffected side; fold a pillow in half and place it behind your back for support. Place another pillow or two under your affected arm. If you like to bend your knees while you sleep, place still another pillow between your knees.

You may find that you are having difficulty getting to sleep at night, and that you are waking up during the night and having trouble falling back to sleep. Sleeping problems can be caused by stress, anxiety, and depression. These feelings are a common and very normal response to diagnosis and treatment. If you haven't done so already, read the section on "Your Emotional Recovery."

If you have any problem sleeping, try the following:

◆ Cut out beverages with caffeine (coffee, tea, carbonated beverages, chocolate) five hours before bedtime.

◆ Take your pain medication twenty minutes before bedtime.

◆ Drink some chamomile tea at bedtime.

◆ Take a warm bath. Just remember not to get your dressing wet or submerge your drain.

◆ Listen to a relaxation tape or practice the relaxation exercise on page 49.

Eating Healthy

Your diet is an important part of your recovery. Eating the right kinds of food after surgery and during your radiation treatment can help you feel better and stay stronger. A nutritious diet is always essential for your body to work most effectively. For people with cancer, good nutrition is especially vital:

◆ A healthy diet can help you keep up your strength, prevent body tissue from breaking down, and rebuild tissues that cancer treatment may harm.

◆ People who eat well during their treatment are better able to cope with the side effects of treatment.

When you are unable to eat enough food or the right kinds of food, your body uses stored nutrients as a source of energy. As a result, your natural defenses (your immune system) are weakened and your body is not as effective in fighting infection. This defense system is especially important to you at this time.

Try to eat a variety of foods every day. No one food or group of foods contains all the nutrients you need. A diet designed to keep your body strong will include daily servings from these food groups:

◆ Fruits and Vegetables: Raw or cooked vegetables, fruits, and fruit juices provide vitamins and minerals the body needs.

◆ Protein: Protein helps your body heal itself and fight infection. Beans, tofu, fish, and poultry (skinless) are low in fat and rich in protein.

◆ Grains: Bread, pasta, and cereals provide carbohydrates and B vitamins. Carbohydrates provide a good source of energy.

Try to drink eight 8-ounce glasses of liquid a day. This is particularly important during radiation therapy and chemotherapy. Drinking liquids flushes out waste products which result from treatment. The following liquids can be included, if tolerated: water, fruit juice, herbal tea, non-caffeinated tonic, and milk.

Beverages that contain caffeine or alcohol are not included in the above list because they are dehydrating. A moderate amount of caffeinated beverages and/or alcohol can be drunk, if you can tolerate them.

Taking Care of Constipation

During the first few days at home, some women find that they are troubled by constipation. Temporary constipation can be the result of anesthesia, pain medication, and/or inactivity. The following are a few suggestions that should get you back to normal and keep you regular:

◆ Drink eight (8) glasses of liquid a day. The following liquids can be included, if tolerated: water, fruit juice, herbal tea, non-caffeinated tonic, and milk. Caffeinated coffee, tea, sodas, and alcohol should not be counted as liquids because they are dehydrating. However, some women find that a cup of coffee or tea in the morning helps bring on a bowel movement.

◆ Increase the fiber in your diet with bran cereals, fruits, and vegetables.

◆ Practice some form of physical activity every day.

◆ Eat prunes or drink prune juice. This also helps you move your bowels.

If you're undergoing chemotherapy, the above suggestions on diet and constipation need some modification. Check under "Treatment" in the *Resource Guide* at the end of the book for information on caring for yourself while under chemotherapy.

*N*ote: The section on nutrition was adapted from a book entitled, *Eating Hints and Recipes and Tips for Better Nutrition During Cancer Treatment.* It can be obtained, free of charge, from the National Institute of Health.

Driving

*Y*ou can begin driving again when you feel ready and when you are no longer taking narcotic pain medication. Turning the wheel and/or parallel parking may feel uncomfortable, but you won't injure your incision when you do so. The type of car you drive (power steering versus manual steering) will also affect how comfortable it is to drive.

Going Back to Work

*G*oing back to work is based on a number of factors and should be decided after a discussion with your doctors. Some important considerations will be: how physically and emotionally demanding and stressful your job is; how much you want to return to work; how fast you are healing; whether you become fatigued from radiation therapy; and whether you are going to need further therapy, such as chemotherapy.

Should you tell your co-workers that you are undergoing treatment for breast cancer? This question is important to consider, not because you should be embarrassed about having breast cancer, but for practical reasons. Under the Federal Rehabilitation Act of 1973, federal employers or companies receiving federal funding cannot discriminate against cancer survivors. But state laws vary, and federal legislation does not affect the private sector.

If your co-workers know your medical history, you may risk overt, as well as more subtle, discrimination. So, some women choose to keep quiet about their diagnosis at work. There is a catch, however. If no one knows about your diagnosis, you can't get the support you may need. This is a difficult situation for which there is no easy answer. You need to do what feels right for you.

5.

Your Exercise Program

Exercise Is Encouraged

*E*xercise reduces stress and fatigue and helps you regain and maintain energy. It's beneficial for both your physical and emotional recovery.

If you have been involved in a strenuous exercise program before surgery, such as running, tennis, aerobics, or weightlifting, you will probably be able to get back to it in about six weeks after your surgery. One qualification is necessary. In three to four weeks after surgery you will begin your radiation treatment or chemotherapy. A common temporary side effect of radiation therapy and chemotherapy is fatigue. So, you may find that you don't have the stamina that you need for strenuous exercise. On the other hand, you may find that you do have the energy. In either case, when you start up again, begin slowly. Before starting or resuming an exercise program, talk with your surgeon and radiation oncologist.

A gentle walking program is beneficial and appropriate, even for a woman who has not exercised for a number of years. Walking every day during your radiation therapy and chemotherapy is a gentle way to stay physically active and may help you sustain your energy.

Exercises to Prepare You for Radiation Therapy

*A*fter surgery, you may notice that your chest, underarm area, and shoulder feel tight and sore on the affected side when you move your arm. In time, you will recover full use of your arm, but you will have to work at regaining arm strength and flexibility. The following six-week exercise program has been designed to get your arm flexibility back to normal and to prepare you for radiation therapy. During radiation therapy you will be asked to lie on a treatment table with your arm extended out to your side, like this.

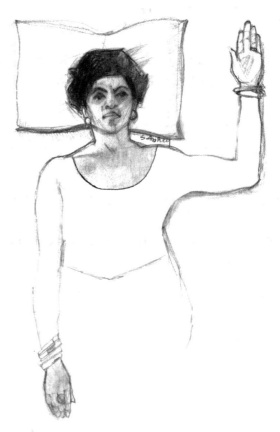

At the end of the second week after surgery, check your arm flexibility by lying on your bed with your arm extended in the position that you will need for radiation therapy. It's important to know that radiation therapy usually starts the third week after surgery, and it may have to be delayed if your arm is not flexible enough.

How Often?

◆ The Arm Pumps and the stretching exercises should be done two times a day, *every day.*

◆ The weightlifting exercises should be done once a day, *every other day.*

◆ The relaxation exercise can be done as often as you find it helpful.

How Much Do I Stretch?

◆ Try to reach farther each time you do the exercise. When you feel your incision pulling, stop and hold the stretch.

◆ Stretching effectively feels uncomfortable (not unbearable). Don't worry. You will not open up your incision.

How Long Do I Hold Each Stretch?

◆ Hold your stretches for at least 15 seconds. Do not bounce when stretching.

The Day After Surgery — Exercise to Reduce Swelling

Arm Pumps

Purpose: To reduce swelling and increase lymphatic drainage start the day after surgery. Perform the exercise throughout your recovery if you notice swelling in your hand and/or your arm.

Position: Sit with your affected arm resting comfortably on pillows. Your arm should be higher than your heart.

Motion: While making a fist, bring your hand toward your shoulder. Then straighten your arm while relaxing your hand. Repeat five times.

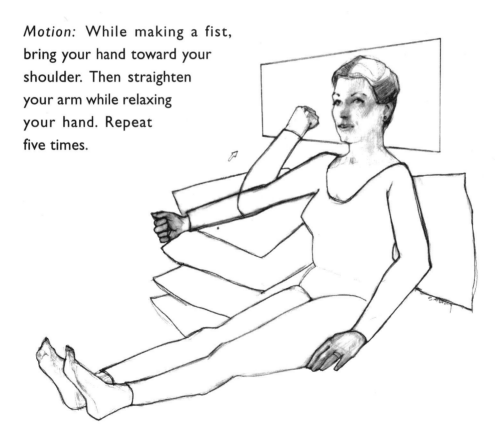

Stretching Exercises

WEEK ONE (WHILE THE DRAIN IS IN)

Arm Raises

Purpose: To keep your shoulder flexible

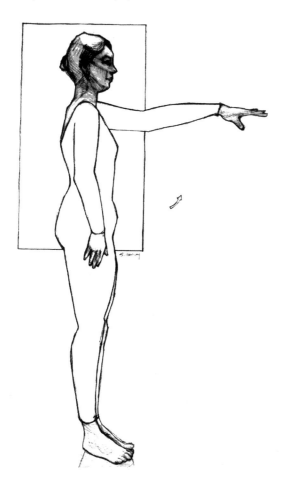

Position: Stand, preferably in front of a mirror, with your arms by your side.

Motion: Keeping your arms straight, slowly raise both arms in front of you to shoulder level. Then, slowly spread both arms out to the side until your arms are parallel to the floor. Lower both arms.

Repeat five times.

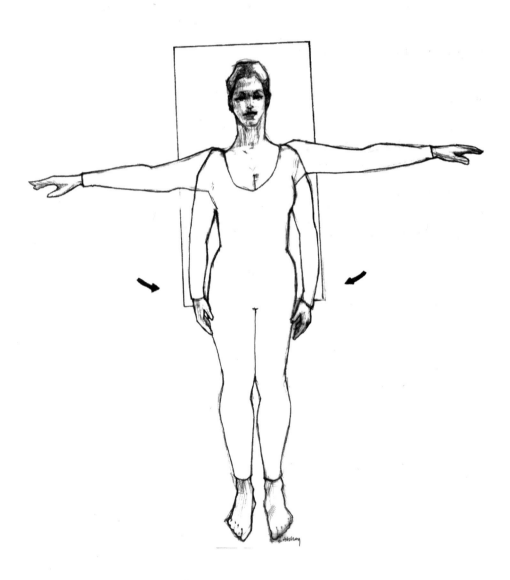

WEEK TWO (AFTER THE DRAIN IS REMOVED)

Clasp-Lift-Stretch

Purpose: To increase the range of motion of your affected arm

Position: Stand

Motion:

1. Clasp your hands together in front of you. Slowly raise your hands toward the ceiling. Make sure your elbows are not bent, and your arms are straight. Stop when you feel your incision pulling. Hold that position for 15 seconds.

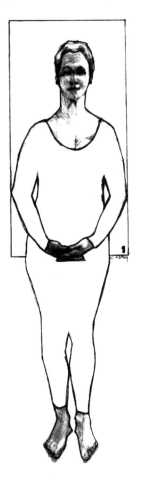
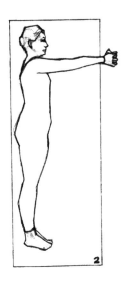

2. With your fingers still clasped, bend your arms and rest your clasped hands on the top of your head. Gradually extend your elbows back. Hold for 15 seconds. Keep your head upright.

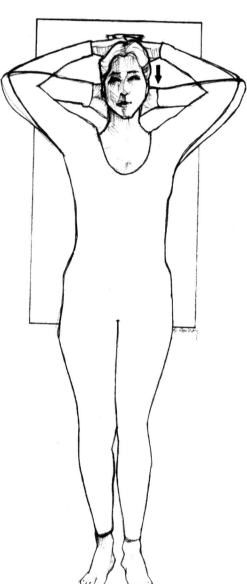

3. As step 2 gets easier, challenge yourself by continuing to slide your clasped hands over your head until you reach the back of your neck. Gradually extend your elbows apart. Hold for 15 seconds. Keep your head upright. Do exercise once.

WEEKS THREE TO SIX

Shoulder Stretch

Purpose: To stretch your underarm and the muscles in the back of your affected arm

Position: Stand facing a wall, with your arm reaching up the wall as far as possible and your palm flat against the wall.

Motion: Lean forward until you feel a stretch in your underarm area. Hold for 15 seconds. As your ability to stretch improves, begin the exercise standing farther away from the wall. Do once.

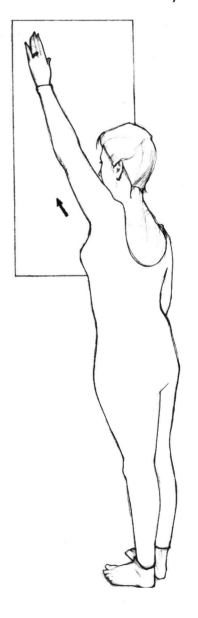

Corner Stretch

Purpose: To stretch the chest muscles

Position: Stand facing a corner. Brace the palms of your hands and fore-arms against the walls on each side of the corner. Keep your elbows at shoulder level.

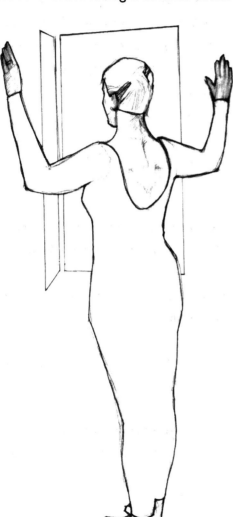

Motion: Slowly lean your chest in toward the corner. Keep your elbows at shoulder level and your forearms flat against the wall throughout the move-ment. You will feel the stretch across your chest wall. Hold this position for 15 seconds. Do once.

Gentle Weightlifting Exercises

WEEKS THREE TO SIX

*T*hese exercises require you to use weights to gently strengthen your arm muscles. Building and keeping your arm muscles strong reduce your risk for lymphedema. Strong arm muscles help the lymphatic drainage system in your arms to work effectively. In addition, having strong arms helps to prevent you from injuring your affected arm.

◆ Start off with one-pound weights and slowly build up to three pounds. (You don't have to buy special equipment; you can use canned goods for your weights.)

◆ Do not exceed three pounds. If you have previously used heavier weights, ask your hospital physical therapist for some guidelines.

◆ Perform these exercises only once a day, *every other day.* Your muscles need a day to repair themselves.

◆ Perform these exercises in front of a mirror so that you can check your form.

It is important to breathe correctly when working with weights. You exhale (breath out) when you work the muscle; you take a deep breath in (inhale) when you relax the muscle.

Shoulder Flexion

Purpose: To work the deltoid muscle, the muscle that allows you to raise the arm overhead

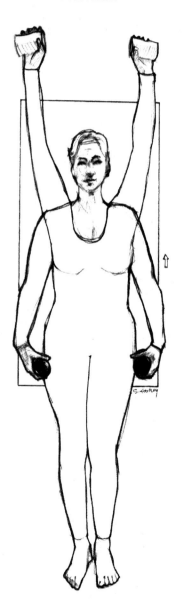

Position: Stand with your arms down by your sides, holding weights.

Motion: Keeping your arms straight, raise both of them over your head directly in front of your body. Exhale as you perform this motion. Inhale as you slowly lower both arms.

Repeat 10 times.

Arm Bending

Purpose: To work the biceps muscle, the muscle that helps you to straighten the arm

Position: Stand with your arms down by your sides, holding weights.

Motion: Bend your arms and bring your hands toward your shoulder. Exhale as you perform this motion. Inhale, as you slowly return to your starting position.

Repeat 10 times.

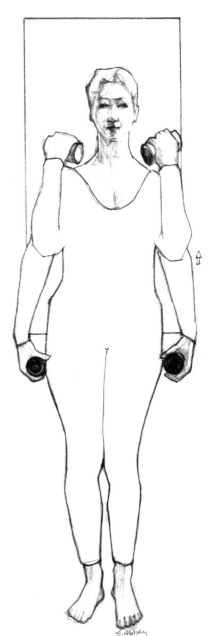

Arm Extension

Purpose: To work the triceps muscle, the muscle that helps you to straighten the arm

Position: Lie on your back with a weight in your affected hand. Bend your arm toward your body so that your elbow points up toward the ceiling. Hold your arm still with your opposite hand.

Motion: Slowly straighten your arm until it is fully extended. Exhale as you perform this motion. Inhale, as you slowly return to your starting position.

Repeat 10 times with each arm.

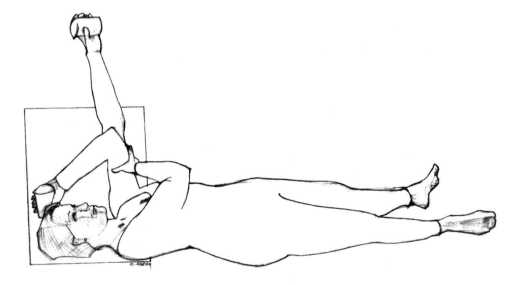

After Six Weeks

After six weeks you are usually able to resume all previous activities. You may choose to do these exercises by yourself or get some professional instruction from a physical therapist. If you feel assistance would help, ask your surgeon for a referral to a physical therapist.

Relaxation Exercise

Do this exercise at the end of your exercise routine, or anytime you want to calm yourself and feel more relaxed. Try this exercise at bedtime to help you fall asleep, or during your radiation treatment to help you relax.

Make Sure That You Are Physically Comfortable

1. If you are hungry, thirsty, or need to go to the bathroom, take care of these needs before you do the relaxation exercise.

2. Find a room that will be conducive to relaxation — a room that is quiet, dimly lit, and at a comfortable temperature.

3. Adjust your clothing so that you are comfortable; for instance, unbutton a tight waistband or collar and remove your shoes.

4. Lie down on a bed, sofa, or the treatment table, or sit on a comfortable chair with both feet touching the floor. Place the palms of your hands on your thighs.

YOUR RELAXATION EXERCISE

Close your eyes. Take a few deep, slow, easy breaths. Think of a time when you felt relaxed and peaceful — perhaps during a walk in the park, a day at the beach, or sitting on your porch. Focus intently on the sights, smells, and physical sensations associated with that event. Focus on this image for at least five minutes. Try to spend a little longer period each time you do this exercise.

When you return to everyday reality, you are likely to feel calm, relaxed, and more refreshed than before — as if you had taken a long rest.

6.

Your Radiation Treatment

....

*R*adiation therapy is an effective, safe way to treat breast cancer. It's needed after a lumpectomy to eliminate any remaining cancer cells in the breast. It's generally well tolerated and most women continue to enjoy an active life during therapy.

Radiation is a kind of energy in the form of invisible waves (x-rays). Special highly technical equipment is used to monitor and precisely aim the radiation at the treatment site. Radiation therapy is most often administered from outside the body (external radiation therapy) using a linear accelerator or cobalt therapy machine. This treatment is provided during outpatient visits to the radiation treatment center, Monday through Friday. Treatments usually take about 15 minutes, with most of the time spent lying down on a treatment table and getting into the correct position. The radiation itself lasts about one minute. A course of external radiation treatments typically lasts five to seven-and-a-half weeks.

Sometimes, radiation therapy is also administered internally. The radiation oncology physician surgically inserts small, sealed, radioactive sources directly into the tumor area. This is usually an inpatient procedure requiring hospitalization for a day or two, until the radioactive sources are removed. More will be said about this procedure on page 61.

Radiation therapy is very effective at killing breast cancer cells. The energy from radiation destroys the ability of cancer cells to function and reproduce, so they die. Normal tissue is also affected by radiation. An irritation or skin redness usually develops a few weeks into treatment. Normal cells, however, recover from the effects of radiation therapy. This means, for example, that after radiation treatments are completed the skin recovers — appears normal again — though the cancer cells have died off.

Except for temporary skin irritation and mild fatigue, side effects during the course of treatment are unusual. Serious and lasting side effects are very rare. Current treatment techniques avoid radiation to the heart. Only a small amount of lung under the treated breast receives radiation. There is very little chance that radiation treatment will cause another cancer.

When you receive radiation treatment, you lie on a table with the radiation equipment directly above you. Many women worry that radiation enters the body through the breast and chest and leaves through the back, penetrating the heart and lungs. This is not what happens. Radiation therapy to your breast is administered at an angle across the surface of your chest. So, your heart and lungs are not involved.

Your Radiation Treatment Team

Radiation therapy is specifically tailored for each patient. It must be carefully planned and calculated. A highly trained health care team of radiation specialists are involved in planning and carrying out your treatment. Your radiation therapy team may include the following:

Your *Radiation Oncologist* heads the team. He or she evaluates your case, and then plans and supervises your treatment. Your doctor will meet with you often during treatment for checkups and address any questions or concerns you may have.

The *Radiation Oncologist Nurse* helps you learn about your treatment, explains how to take care of yourself during treatment, and teaches you how to manage any possible side effects. She is also an excellent source of information about resources and services in the hospital and in the community, such as support groups and transportation to and from treatment.

The *Radiation Therapists* or *Technologists* administer your daily treatment. They begin by placing you in the right position on the treatment table. Then the therapists start the treatment. They monitor the machine until the radiation being administered is stopped at the prescribed dose.

The *Radiation Physicist* maintains the radiation equipment. He makes sure that the equipment is working properly, so that the treatment machine delivers exactly the right dose of radiation to precisely the right area.

The *Dosimetrist* works with the doctor, the physicist, and the therapist to plan and calculate the daily and overall treatment dose.

These, then, are the primary members of your radiation therapy team. However, you may see other health care professionals during the course of your treatment, such as a dietitian, a physical therapist, or a social worker.

An Overview of Your Radiation Treatment

Your radiation therapy involves careful evaluation and planning to calculate the exact dose and proper placement of the radiation. You will first meet your doctor, the radiation oncologist, for a medical evaluation and to have answered any questions you may have. The first consultation with your doctor is followed by a special appointment to plan your daily treatment. It is called a *simulation* appointment.

As mentioned, radiation therapy is usually given five days a week for five to eight weeks. The treatment itself lasts about one minute. You'll be in the treatment room for about 10 to 15 minutes and in the radiation department less than an hour each day. The appointment time is usually the same each day, so if you prefer to come in at particular time during the day, an effort will be made to accommodate you.

As said, your first appointment is a consultation with your radiation oncologist. Your doctor will perform a careful breast and physical examination, and will review your medical history. The rest of the appointment will be spent explaining the treatment, reviewing the risks and benefits of the treatment, and answering your questions. You are encouraged to bring up any of your questions or concerns. It may be helpful for you to review the section in the book called "Talking to Your Doctor" on page 5. Below are some questions you may want to ask:

◆ How long will the daily treatments last?

◆ How long will I be in the radiation therapy department?

◆ How many weeks will the treatment take?

◆ What are the risks and benefits?

◆ What are the common short-term side effects?

◆ What are the common long-term side effects?

◆ What can be done to reduce the side effects?

◆ How often will I need to see you after treatment ends?

Your Simulation Appointment

*T*he radiation therapy team will need to do special planning to exactly pinpoint the treatment area. Your general treatment area is the whole breast, from just below your collarbone to below your breast and from your underarm to your breastbone. Sometimes the lymph nodes above the collarbone are also treated. However, the treatment area must be much more precisely pinpointed. As said, particular effort is made to avoid giving radiation to your heart and your lungs. The planning begins with a special session called *simulation*.

A simulation appointment will be made for you after you meet with you radiation oncology doctor and a few days before you are scheduled to begin treatment. During simulation, you will be asked to lie on a table while the doctor and radiation therapist outline, on your skin, the specific treatment area. X-ray pictures are then taken to check the position of your body and to see the internal areas of your body, such as your heart and lungs.

This appointment is one of the longest sessions you will have during treatment. It can last from one to two hours. Remember, you will only be in the treatment room for about fifteen minutes during the actual radiation treatment.

Because exact measurements must be taken, your radiation therapist will ask you to relax, breath normally, and lie very still during the simulation. It is important that you plan your day so that you allow enough time for your appointment, which will last approximately two hours. Try to arrive early and try not to schedule anything directly after the appointment. That way, you won't feel rushed or tense about time.

When you arrive for your simulation appointment, you'll be asked to undress from the waist up and to put on a hospital gown. You'll be taken to a simulation or treatment room and asked to lie down on a table. A large x-ray machine (the simulator) will be above you. Some women find that the machine looks scary, while others are fascinated by it and say that it looks like something out of "Star Trek."

One of the first things that is done is that a "mold" or an "immobility device" is made for your back and arm on the affected side. This device will be used during all your treatments to cradle your back and arm in exactly the same position each time and to minimize movement.

Different materials can be used to make the mold. An Alpha Cradle is made of liquid styrofoam. It takes about 15 minutes to set and feels warm against your body. Some women describe it as feeling soothing and comforting. Another type of mold is called a VAC Bag. This mold is filled with air. Still another device is called a Breast Board and is made of lucite.

While the mold or treatment device is being prepared, it's important that you do not move, that you relax your torso and breath normally. Remember the relaxation exercise on page 49.

After the treatment device is made, you'll remain in the treatment position for the rest of the simulation procedure. It is then that the radiation therapists will start taking measurements of the treatment site. They will make subtle changes in the position of your body. They will change the position of the simulator several times. As it moves, it will make a buzzing noise. Remember to lie still and breath normally.

During the simulation, your doctor and radiation therapist will outline the treatment area on your skin, often with semi-permanent ink. Sometimes, very tiny black or blue permanent tattoo dots are placed on your chest. You may be asked not to wash the ink off. However, it is all right to take a shower, just don't wash with soap over these areas. Pat rather than rub yourself dry with a towel. (A word of caution, the ink can stain your clothes.)

The simulation appointment can be uncomfortable because you are asked to lie still for such a long time. Some women feel "antsy" toward the end. Your hand and arm may fall asleep and feel numb. Your shoulder may become stiff and feel tight and uncomfortable. Just remember, these feelings are temporary! At the end of the simulation, your shoulder and arm will relax when you begin to move them again. The following may help you relax during stimulation:

1. Allow yourself enough time for the appointment so that you don't feel rushed.

2. Don't drink more than one cup of coffee or black tea before your appointment since stimulants may make you more tense. Drinking chamomile tea may help you relax.

3. Listening to music through a tape player headset is helpful for some people during the simulation.

4. Try to relax and think positive, healthy thoughts. Perform the relaxation exercise on page 49.

After the simulation is over, your radiation oncologist and dosimetist or physicist work together to fine-tune the preparation for your actual treatment. Your radiation oncologist decides how much radiation is needed, how it will be delivered, and how many treatments you should have. This process usually takes two to four days.

Your Treatment Visits

*B*efore you begin your treatment, you will be asked to undress from the waist up and change into a hospital gown. You will be taken to the treatment room and asked to lie down on the treatment table. Like the simulation equipment, the radiation therapy equipment is quite large and may seem scary at first. If you feel concerned or have *any* questions, talk with the radiation therapists. They will make every effort to see that you feel safe and comfortable. Your individualized treatment cradle will be placed under your back and arm. Then, the radiation therapists will carefully position your body and the machine. This may take up to 10 minutes.

While the machine is being positioned, it will make a noise. This noise doesn't mean that radiation is being emitted. You'll be asked to lie very still during this time. This may be tedious, but it's necessary, to make sure that the radiation is directed to exactly the right area.

After your therapists determine that your body and the machine are positioned perfectly, the radiation therapists will leave the room and begin your treatment. The treatment continues for about a minute and is completely painless, much like taking a chest x-ray.

After the desired dosage has been administered, the machine will turn off automatically. You'll receive radiation therapy from two different angled directions. Your therapists will come back into the treatment room to reposition the machine and your body for the other direction. Again, your therapist will leave the room and the treatment will continue for several more seconds.

As mentioned, you will need to remain very still during the treatment. Remember, the treatment lasts for about a minute. You don't have to hold your breath — just breathe normally. You may want to close your eyes and take slow breaths which may help you relax. Some women like to visualize that the radiation is sending a healing energy into their bodies.

Although you may feel alone, you are not. Your radiation therapist will be watching you on a television screen or through a window during your whole treatment. You can also talk to your therapist through a speaker during your treatment.

When the daily treatment is over, your therapist will come back into the room. You'll then be able to get up, get dressed, and leave. You should feel fine. If you have any questions or concerns, make sure you talk to the radiation nurse. Once a week, either before or after your treatment, you'll meet with your radiation doctor, who will check your progress and answer any of your questions and concerns.

Radiation Boost

Sometimes, after you've completed your course of treatment, additional radiation is administered to a smaller area, the area where the tumor used to be or where the lumpectomy was done. This is called a *radiation boost* and is intended to eliminate any cancer cells that might remain around the lumpectomy area. The radiation boost is commonly administered externally. In some treatment centers, it is dispensed through internal radiation. The type of boost given largely depends on the equipment the hospital has.

When you receive your external radiation boost treatment, you probably won't notice any difference in your treatment routine. You'll be treated in the same department and in a similar way as when you received your regular treatments. The only difference is that the radiation therapist will adjust the radiation equipment so that the field of radiation is smaller. External radiation boost treatments are often given by electron beam therapy, which is a beam of subatomic particles. This is a less penetrating form of radiation than the x-ray, so you needn't be concerned that your heart or lungs will receive radiation. The radiation boost treatments are generally administered daily, for one to three weeks.

Internal Radiation

Sometimes, radiation boosts are administered through internal radiation using a radioactive implant. Internal radiation is a simple and safe inpatient procedure by which a radioactive implant is placed in the breast around the area of the tumor. You'll stay in the hospital for a day or two, while the radiation material is in your breast.

The first part of the procedure requires the insertion of several very small tubes (without the radioactive material in them) into your breast. This is performed in an operating room by your radiation oncologist, either at the time of your lumpectomy or in a separate procedure at the end of radiation therapy. Since this is a fairly simple procedure, a local anesthesia can be used. Sometimes a general anesthesia is used.

After the insertion of the tubes, you will be brought to a private hospital room where your radiation oncologist will place a small amount of radioactive material into the tubes. There is generally no pain with this procedure. Sometimes, you may feel some slight discomfort. Once the radioactive material is in place, you will be asked to remain in your hospital room until the radioactive material is removed.

The radioactive substance in your implant may transmit radioactive rays into the area around your body. Other than the very small area where the implant is placed, your body will not receive a significant amount of radiation. You needn't be concerned about any ill effects on your body.

However, since the hospital staff works around radiation every day, an effort is made to reduce the amount of accumulated radiation they receive. So, while your implant is in place, the hospital will limit the amount of time that nurses and others who care for you spend with you each day. They will provide for all of your required care, but expect your nurses and the other staff to work quickly and to speak to you from the doorway more often than from your bedside.

The hospital will also place limits on visitors. Children under 18 or pregnant women will not be allowed to visit you. Visitors will be asked to sit at least six feet from your bed and to limit their stay to less than one hour each day.

You will be able to care for yourself, just fine. You'll feel normal, without pain or discomfort, and will be able to move around the room freely. You'll be able to take care of your grooming needs, although you will be asked not to take a shower or to get your implant wet.

Although you'll feel fine physically, you may become a little bored and lonely. Since you will be in the hospital for about one to three days, without much company, you may want to bring along some things to pass the time:

◆ Cassette player and some favorite tapes

◆ Books and magazines

◆ Crafts, such as knitting or needlepoint

◆ Crossword and jigsaw puzzles

After the completion of your internal radiation boost treatment, your radiation oncologist will come into your room and remove the radioactive material and the tubes from your breast. Usually, there is no need to have anesthesia for the removal of the implant. After the radioactive material has been removed, it's perfectly safe for you to hold even an infant.

Managing Side Effects

Radiation therapy is generally well tolerated. It causes only mild, temporary side effects and generally will not interfere with your daily activities. Many women are able to go to work, keep house, and enjoy leisure activities while they are receiving radiation therapy. The most common temporary side effects are fatigue and some skin changes. If these develop, they usually go away in a few weeks after the treatment ends. Radiation therapy to your breast won't cause you to lose your hair, become nauseous, or affect your blood. Nor will you be radioactive. After your daily treatment, it is perfectly safe to hug, even the smallest child.

Before beginning your treatment, ask your doctor and nurse to review any possible side effects. Here are some of questions you might ask:

◆ What are the possible side effects?

◆ How long will they last?

◆ How serious will they be?

◆ Is there something I can do to reduce the side effects?

MANAGING FATIGUE

During radiation therapy the body uses a lot of energy healing itself. Stress related to your illness, daily trips for treatment, and the temporary, damaging effects of radiation on normal cells may all contribute to fatigue.

Most people begin to feel tired after a few weeks of radiation therapy. Fatigue may last from four to six weeks after your treatment is finished.

You can help yourself during radiation therapy by setting priorities. Decide what is *really* important for you to do, what others can help you with, and what you should let go of. Try to let go of activities and responsibilities that are physically and emotionally draining.

If you work at a full-time job, you may want or need to continue working. However, some women prefer to take a few weeks off from work while they are receiving radiation therapy; others work a reduced number of hours. You may want to speak with your employer about your needs and wishes during this time. You may be able to agree on a part-time schedule; maybe you can do some work at home. The following may keep your energy up:

◆ Ask a family member or friend to help with daily chores, shopping, child care, housework, or driving.

◆ Good nutrition is important. Try to eat a balanced diet. (Page 30)

◆ Drink plenty of liquids. Eight glasses of non-caffeinated liquids a day will prevent dehydration that can contribute to fatigue. Also, water helps the body eliminate the waste products that can build up during treatment. (Page 32)

◆ Do some routine daily exercise during treatment. Regular exercise can help you maintain your energy. (Page 35)

◆ Practice some form of relaxation exercise. Stress can make you feel more tired. Relaxation exercises can reduce stress and give you more energy. (Page 49)

◆ Try to get some extra sleep at night. Nap during the day if needed. (Page 29)

SKIN CHANGES

Radiation therapy causes temporary sunburn-like changes in your skin. Around the third week of treatment you may notice that the skin in the treatment area may begin to look red, irritated, or tanned. You may develop dry skin over the treated area. Women who are heavier and have skin folds may develop some blisters in those folds.

Mild lotions are recommended to help heal the skin and to reduce discomfort. Your nurse or doctor will give you specific information about a special lotion or skin cream to use. Gently apply the lotion to the whole treated area: from the middle of your underarm to your breastbone (sternum) and from your lower bra line up to your collarbone. Also, include your shoulder and upper back. Apply the lotion after your treatment, after your bath or shower, and at bedtime. Start the first day of treatment and continue throughout.

Different products work better on different women. It may be helpful to try another product if you're not getting a good result from the one you're using. Always ask your doctor or nurse before applying any product on your skin. Many skin products can leave a coating on the skin that can interfere with radiation therapy or healing. For those who develop blisters, you'll be given a special dressing to apply to the skin that encourages rapid healing.

During radiation therapy you will need to be very gentle with the skin over the treated area. Think of your skin as having a sunburn. That way you'll know how to take care of it — what you should do and what you should avoid.

Things to Do

◆ Go without a bra whenever possible. If this is not possible, wear a soft, loose, cotton bra without underwires. Make sure the cup is not too tight, since your breast may swell slightly.

◆ Wear soft, loose, comfortable clothing next to your skin.

◆ Gently apply a recommended lotion to the whole treated area, twice a day, throughout your treatment.

◆ If your skin itches, apply refrigerated cornstarch. Pat areas that itch, very gently. Don't scratch the area!

◆ Use cool water when you wash the treated area.

Things to Avoid on the Treatment Area

◆ Avoid using soap, as they dry the skin. If you must use soap, use a super fatty soap, such as Bases or unscented Dove.

◆ Don't wear tight clothing over the treated area.

◆ Do not rub, scrub, or scratch the skin.

◆ Avoid putting anything that is very hot on the area, such as a heating pad. Avoid hot tubs or saunas.

◆ Avoid putting anything very cold on the area, such as an ice pack.

◆ Don't apply anything to the skin (powders, creams, perfumes, body oils) unless specially recommended.

◆ Don't shave your underarm. If you must shave, use an electric razor.

◆ Avoid using deodorants.

◆ Avoid exposing the area to the sun during treatment.

◆ For about a year after your treatment is completed, avoid exposing the treated area to the sun. When in the sun, always wear protective clothing and sunblocking lotions that are recommended by your doctor or nurse.

LONG-TERM SIDE EFFECTS

After treatment is over, a few women experience some long-term side effects. Some women find that their breast feels different. Occasional soreness or moments of needle-like sensations may occur for months — or even years — after treatment. Slowly, over time, the discomfort will diminish.

The skin of the nipple and areola (the dark area surrounding the nipple) may feel slightly firmer. When you perform breast self-examination you may notice that your breast feels slightly firmer to the touch, and smoother, less lumpy, upon deeper examination.

Sometimes, a small fracture develops in a rib on the side that was treated. The fracture can cause discomfort when you press your breast. The tiny fracture is not dangerous and it does not have to be treated. It heals on its own in a few months.

Your breast will probably look the same. If changes do occur they usually will be slight. For instance, the pores might be larger; your breast may be slightly smaller or larger; your breast may appear more uplifted.

At the End of Your Treatment

You may find that you face the end of treatment with mixed emotions. During treatment, most women feel safe — that their cancer is actively and effectively being treated. After treatment ends, you may feel a little scared. You may also feel a little sad to leave the supportive atmosphere of the radiation department and the daily caring support of your radiation therapy team.

But remember, your team is still there for you. After treatment ends, your doctor will be happy to address any question or concern that you may have at your routine check-up or during a telephone call between appointments. This may also be a time, if you have not done so already, to join a support group. A support group provides understanding, strength, and companionship. Finally, you can take away from your treatment the assurance that lumpectomy combined with radiation therapy is a strong, safe, and effective treatment for breast cancer.

7.

Your Emotional Recovery

Taking Care of Your Feelings

You will need to make your own needs and feelings your top priority during the course of your diagnosis, treatment, and recovery. Though this may sound obvious, it may be difficult to do. Many women are used to putting other people's needs — those of children, partners, friends — ahead of their own. Women who easily help others find it difficult to ask for help for themselves. Yet, taking care of yourself by reaching out to people who can provide you with support is essential to getting well. Your emotional recovery should be as consciously pursued as your physical recovery.

Be kind to yourself. Treat yourself to activities that make you feel good and give you pleasure. They don't necessarily have to cost a lot of money. Walking in the park, sitting on your porch, taking care of your plants or garden, relaxing in a warm bath, or getting a massage can be very comforting. Try to let go of activities and responsibilities that are physically and emotionally draining. Set priorities. Do those things that give you satisfaction; try to let go of the "oughts" and "shoulds."

Be honest with yourself. In order to receive support from others, you need to know what you want and need from them. This is a time to look inward; it's a time to explore your feelings, needs, and desires. Then, you must have the strength to communicate those needs and feelings in as direct and honest a manner as possible.

Selecting Your Support Team

SEEK OUT FAMILY AND FRIENDS

*F*amily and friends can be a wonderful source of support and help. However, sometimes they don't know what to say or do. Help them comfort you.

◆ Let them know they don't have to say anything; all they need to do is just be there — to sit with you, to listen to you, to let you cry.

◆ Ask them to help with meals, to run errands, to care for your children, to drive you, or to come with you to appointments. Some people feel more comfortable showing their support by "doing" rather than talking or listening.

Not everyone is able to give you the support and understanding you need in the way that you need it. Some of your co-workers, friends, and family, no matter how well-meaning, can make you feel worse rather than better. Sometimes, some of your friends or relatives may become cold or distant when you tell them about your breast cancer. In extreme cases, they may literally disappear from your life. Often, they have an irrational fear of cancer. Although their absence may be very painful to you, and it may feel like a personal rejection, remember, they are reacting to their fear of cancer, not to their feelings about you.

JOIN A SUPPORT GROUP

A strong remedy for dealing with painful experiences is to be able to talk to others who are going through similar experiences. During treatment and recovery, it's particularly helpful to talk with other women who have breast cancer. Most of them, like yourself, have experienced a range of strong and often scary emotions such as fear, depression, and anger. Seeing others express emotions similar to yours will help you realize that your own feelings are normal.

A support group provides understanding, strength, and companionship; it becomes a safe place to express feelings that you can't or won't share with family or friends. Whether you have family or not, the group becomes a "family" of special friends.

Each support group has its own personality — made unique by the women who participate in it. If you go to a support group meeting and it isn't a good fit, don't be discouraged. Try another support group; it's worth it. Many women feel that their support group is vital to their emotional recovery.

To find a support group, ask your doctors, nurse, or hospital social worker for leads, or call some of the organizations listed in the *Resource Guide.*

FIND ONE-TO-ONE SUPPORT

You may feel most comfortable talking with another breast cancer survivor in a one-to-one situation. One source to which you can turn is the American Cancer Society's "Reach for Recovery" program. The program provides emotional support and information through trained volunteers who have had breast cancer surgery. If you wish, a volunteer can call or visit you at the hospital or at your home. To get in touch with a volunteer, call your local chapter of the American Cancer Society.

Another way to get in touch with a breast cancer survivor is to talk with your doctors, hospital social worker, or clergy about putting you in contact with someone. If there are women's organizations or breast cancer advocacy groups in your city or town, you might want to check with them for referrals.

CONSIDER PROFESSIONAL EMOTIONAL SUPPORT

Sometimes, talking with your family, friends, or support group may not be enough. At such times, talking with a caring mental health professional can be very helpful, since they are specifically trained to focus on your needs. Having private and confidential conversations with a trained professional can help you sort out issues around self-esteem, your feelings about the changes in your body, and your anxiety and fears — really any personal issues that concern you. They can also provide expert guidance on ways to cope with issues and problems that come up with your partner, children, friends, and family.

You can consult with a variety of resource people: for personal concerns, a clinical psychologist, nurse therapist, clinical social worker, or psychiatrist; for marital and family issues, a marriage and family counselor; for sexual concerns, a certified sexual counselor. Ask your doctors and hospital social worker for referrals.

TALK WITH YOUR CHILDREN

You may be tempted to protect your children, and maybe yourself, by not telling them about your diagnosis. However, children — even very young children — can sense when something is wrong. Usually it's better to be honest and involve your children in your recovery process from the beginning. Tell them the truth — simply and in a manner and language appropriate to their age level.

How do you know what is age appropriate? You'll find out by encouraging questions from them. Your children will ask you what they need to know, when they are ready to know it. Give them the information they ask for, not more.

Children absorb stressful information in stages. After they have had time to internalize the information you've given them, they will ask more questions when they are ready. Give your children permission to ask any question. Explain that it's more scary when they don't ask, because their imagination fills in the gaps. If you want some help talking with your children, ask your doctors, your child's doctor, or hospital social worker to set up a consultation with a health care professional who works specifically with children, and who can speak to you alone or meet with you and your family.

Physical and Sexual Intimacy

Resuming, maintaining, or starting a satisfying sexual relationship is an important part of your emotional recovery. Breast surgery can cause a woman to doubt her attractiveness and a loving touch can go a long way toward helping a woman regain sexual self-confidence.

You may not be ready for sexual intimacy, but you may want and need to be touched and hugged without the pressure to go further. Sometimes, even without noticing it, couples drift apart physically; they stop their loving routines, such as cuddling in front of the television or hugging each other.

Notice if this is happening between you and your partner. If it is, make sure to get touch back into your relationship. Holding hands, asking for or giving a hug, or stroking an arm or back all "remind" you and your partner how important you are to each other.

Sometimes, a neck and back massage is also very comforting and an intimate experience that can bring pleasure to both of you, without any pressure to go further. To make the massage more comfortable, you can either lie on your unaffected side or sit up. Use lotion or oil, and warm it by rubbing it between the palms of the hands.

You may find that both you and your partner have less interest in sex than you did before your diagnosis. This is quite common and normal. The stress of diagnosis and treatment, along with the many strong emotions you're probably feeling, can reduce sexual desire. It's difficult to feel romantic when you and your partner are trying to cope with anger, fear, depression, anxiety, and other strong feelings. Talking about these feelings can encourage intimacy; and intimacy can create romance and sexual interest.

In time, you should find your sexual desire returning to the level it was before diagnosis. If your interest isn't returning, ask the doctor with whom you feel most comfortable for a referral to a counselor specially trained to talk with you about sexual intimacy. A certified sex therapist can help you figure out the causes of low sexual desire and suggest steps that can lead to improved sexual satisfaction.

RESUMING YOUR SEXUAL RELATIONS

Resuming your sexual relations may be intimidating. There may be some awkward moments. As with all other aspects of your emotional recovery, it's important for you to be honest with yourself about your needs, concerns, and fears, and to be able to talk with your partner about them.

Sometimes misunderstandings and hurt feelings may develop. For example, your partner may assume you shouldn't have sex for some time after surgery or during radiation, or that you may be "radioactive" during radiation therapy. You partner may also be hesitant for fear that lovemaking will hurt you, which you, in turn, may misinterpret as rejection.

You can prevent these potential misunderstandings by talking frankly with your partner. You can reassure your partner that with a little extra care, love-making won't hurt your breast and that it isn't bad for your health. Your partner can reassure you that you are still loved and desired.

Whenever you and your partner feel ready to have sexual relations, you may find the following helpful:

◆ Wear something that makes you feel comfortable and desirable, like a pretty camisole, nightie, or negligee.

◆ Your incisions may be numb or particularly sensitive to touch. They and your breast may be tender to touch. Some women don't enjoy having their treated breast or the area over the incisions caressed; others do. It's important to let your partner know this — and whatever else — does and doesn't feel good.

◆ There is no right or wrong position for having sex. Whatever position is comfortable for you is the "right" one. Women report that one of the most comfortable positions is with their partner on top. This position puts the least amount of pressure on the breast or incisions, especially if partners use their arms to support themselves.

◆ Try lying with your affected arm over your affected breast, so that your hand is resting on your unaffected shoulder. You can also place a small pillow over your breast. This may help you feel your breast is safe and will allow you to relax.

◆ Tamoxifen, chemotherapy, and/or menopause may cause vaginal dryness. This can interfere with sexual enjoyment. There are a number of good non-prescription products you can buy to provide vaginal lubrication, for example, Replense, Probe, and Astroglide. Replense is good because it is routinely applied and need not be timed with intercourse. It should be applied once in the morning, three times a week. Probe and Astroglide are used as lubricants during intercourse.

You may find that talking to your partner about sex is not easy to do. You're not alone. Many find it difficult to talk openly about sexual matters. If you're having difficulty, a specially trained and certified sex therapist can be of great help. Ask any of your doctors, your hospital social worker, or your personal counselor for a referral.

Tips for Talking About Sexual Intimacy

◆ Set aside a time to talk with each other about sexual intimacy.

◆ Find a time when there are no distractions, the television is off, the children are asleep — time for just the two of you.

◆ Talk with each other in a sexually "neutral" area, not in a place where you are sexually intimate.

◆ Try to talk with each other honestly and with humor.

SINGLE WOMEN AND SEXUAL INTIMACY

*I*f you are a single woman, you may have some special concerns about physical intimacy. One concern you may have is when and how to tell friends and lovers that you have been diagnosed with cancer and have had breast surgery. It can be helpful to talk to other single women who have had breast cancer to find out how they coped, as well as to receive and give emotional support. Ask your friends, hospital social worker, doctors, clergy, and the "Reach for Recovery" coordinator to put you in touch with other single women. There are two books that address the particular concerns of single women. *Up Front: Sex and the Post-Mastectomy Woman* by Linda Dackman is about a woman who had a mastectomy rather than a lumpectomy; nonetheless, it's a helpful book. It is an honest, intimate, and funny account of a single woman living and loving with breast cancer. The other book is *Invisible Scars* by Mimi Greenberg, Ph.D.

Whether you are single or have a partner, it's important to know what you do and don't want and need for yourself. This knowledge will ease recovery for you and for those who love you.

8.

Your Treatment Plan

....

No Further Treatment

*A*fter a lumpectomy and radiation therapy, some women need no further treatment. However, careful follow-up is important. That means regular clinical examinations and mammograms. Below are some of the questions you will need to ask your surgeon and radiation oncologist:

◆ How often do I need to return for examinations?

◆ How often do I need to have a mammogram?

◆ What other kinds of tests do I need to have, and how often do they need to be done?

Other Treatments

*Y*our doctors may suggest the use of other forms of treatment in addition to your lumpectomy and radiation therapy. These may include taking tamoxifen and undergoing chemotherapy. To find out what is the best personal treatment, you should to talk to a medical oncologist, a doctor who treats cancer with medication.

The decision to have further treatment can be a difficult one for you and your doctors to make. Various factors need to be taken into account. Tests, such as a bone scan, chest x-rays, and blood work, may also be needed to make that decision. Just as important are your feelings about undergoing further treatment. These feelings and concerns should be carefully discussed with your doctors.

Some of the factors considered in making a treatment decision include the following:

◆ Tumor size: the size of the cancer in the breast

◆ Lymph node status: the presence or absence of cancer cells in the lymph nodes under the arm on the side of the lumpectomy

◆ Histology: the type of breast cancer it is, and whether it is slow or fast-growing

◆ Hormone assay tests: whether the tumor is receptive to the hormones estrogen and progesterone

◆ DNA analysis: computer analysis of the chromosome content of the tumor to determine whether the cancer is slow or fast-growing

◆ Your own thoughts and feelings: how you feel about further treatment and the nature and effects of that treatment

At first, these tests and their results may seem a bit technical. But don't be put off. If you're interested, your surgeon, medical oncologist, or oncology nurse will be happy to carefully explain what these tests mean in terms of your treatment. In addition, there are a number of good books and pamphlets that explain the nature of these tests in a clear and under-standable manner. *Dr. Susan Love's Breast Book* by Susan M. Love, M.D., is particularly helpful.

Hormonal Therapy

Tamoxifen (Novadex) is the most common oral medication that is given to reduce the risk of the cancer coming back. Tamoxifen treats your whole body — it's *systemic therapy*. Tamoxifen is "hormonal therapy." It's useful to think of tamoxifen as an "anti-estrogen."

To understand how tamoxifen works, it's important to know that some breast cancers "like" estrogen. These cancers are *estrogen receptor positive* tumors so estrogen can encourage the cancer cells to divide and multiply. A woman's body makes estrogen both before and after menopause; of course, after menopause, her body produces less estrogen. When a woman takes tamoxifen, the drug "attaches" itself to cancer cells that may be in the body, and prevents the natural estrogen a woman makes from encouraging the cancer cells to divide. In this way, and pos-sibly in other ways, tamoxifen inhibits the cancer cells from growing.

Tamoxifen is generally well tolerated. Although tamoxifen doesn't cause menopause, it may bring on menopausal symptoms such as hot flashes, night sweats, and vaginal dryness. Some women report experiencing weight gain and depression. While taking tamoxifen, you should get a yearly pap smear and pelvic examination, since there is a slight increase in the risk of developing uterine cancer. For information on managing menopausal symptoms without estrogen replacement therapy, refer to the *Resource Guide* under "Menopause." Tamoxifen is prescribed and monitored either by your surgeon or medical oncologist. Here are some questions you may want to ask these doctors:

◆ What are the risks and benefits of taking tamoxifen?

◆ What are some of the possible side effects of tamoxifen?

◆ How long do I need to take it?

◆ How often do I need to have a pap smear and pelvic examination?

◆ Do I need any other tests on a regular basis if I take tamoxifen?

Chemotherapy

Chemotherapy is a cancer treatment using medication that kills cancer cells (cytotoxic). It's a systemic therapy designed to kill cancer cells that may be in the body. Chemotherapy utilizes a combination of medications that can be given orally and/or intravenously. The medications are given on a set schedule: every few weeks, often for four to six months. The timing of chemotherapy varies. Most often, it is administered after radiation therapy is completed. It may sometimes be given after surgery and before radiation is started. Chemotherapy can be administered on an outpatient basis or during a hospital stay. A medical oncologist plans and supervises chemotherapy.

Most women are surprised to find that conventional chemotherapy is not as bad as they feared it would be. With improved ways of administering it and new anti-nausea medications, nausea and vomiting are the exception, not the rule. Women typically say that they feel "queasy," "out of sorts," and "tired," for about three days after chemotherapy. However, many women feel well enough to work during their course of chemotherapy.

The most obvious outward effect of chemotherapy is a temporary one: hair thinning or hair loss. With some experimentation with hats, scarves, hair pieces, jewelry, and a little makeup, a woman can feel confident and attractive during this time. For information that addresses appearance and chemotherapy, look under "Appearance" in the *Resource Guide*. Other side effects, which are temporary, include fatigue and low blood counts.

Another effect of chemotherapy is that it can cause the onset of menopause and menopausal symptoms, such as hot flashes and vaginal dryness. For information on managing menopausal symptoms without hormone replacement therapy, refer to the *Resource Guide* under "Menopause."

Some women report a lessening of sexual desire — either temporary or permanent. After the completion of chemotherapy, give yourself several months to regain interest in sex. If it doesn't return to what it was before diagnosis, ask the doctor with whom you feel most comfortable for a referral to a counselor specially trained to talk with you about sexual intimacy. A certified sex therapist can help you figure out the cause(s) of low sexual desire. They can help you sort out emotional issues and/or physical issues, such as low testosterone levels, and suggest steps that can lead to enhanced sexual desire.

Your medical oncologist and oncology nurse are sensitive to fears you may have about chemotherapy and will work with you to manage side effects. In addition, there are books on coping with chemotherapy that cover diet, exercise, and relaxation techniques. These resources can help you look and feel your best. See the *Resource Guide* under "Treatment."

Once you are referred to a medical oncologist, there are a number of questions you may want to ask:

◆ What medications do you suggest?

◆ How effective are these drugs in cases similar to mine?

◆ What are the risks and benefits?

◆ How long will I be on chemotherapy?

◆ How often do I come in for treatments?

◆ When will I receive chemotherapy, before or after radiation therapy?

◆ What are the common side effects of chemotherapy?

◆ What can be done to reduce the side effects?

◆ Will I be able to work while on chemotherapy?

◆ How often will I need to see you after treatment ends?

Tips for Coping with Chemotherapy

◆ Get information about taking care of yourself while on chemotherapy. Talk to your oncology nurse, doctor, or women in your support group. Refer to the *Resource Guide* under "Treatment" for recommended books.

◆ Drink plenty of liquids (8 to 10 glasses), particularly the day before, the day of, and the day after chemotherapy. Read page 32 for information on the right types of liquids.

◆ If you're experiencing nausea or vomiting, do not suffer in silence. Talk to your doctor or oncology nurse. You may not be taking your anti-nausea medication correctly, or you may need another type of medication.

Regular Follow-Up

After your treatment ends, you will have frequent clinical examinations and routine mammograms. During the first two years, you will see your doctors every three to six months. Since you may have several doctors — for example, a surgeon, a radiation oncologist, a medical oncologist, and your primary doctor — you will need to check with each to see whom you will visit, and when.

The time after treatment ends and between doctors' visits can be an anxious one. Having gone through a diagnosis of breast cancer and post-surgery treatment, it's no wonder that any physical discomfort you have, such as a headache or a cough, might cause you to be anxious and to have thoughts of a recurrence. The best way to assure yourself that you're okay is to discuss your observations and concerns with your doctors.

Breast Self-Examination

In addition to having clinical breast examinations by your health care provider and regular mammograms, you're encouraged to perform a monthly breast self-examination (BSE).

How to Do BSE

If you continue to menstruate, the best time to do BSE is seven to ten days after the first day of your cycle. This is the time during your menstrual cycle when the breasts are least tender to touch. Remember, if you had pre-menstrual breast tenderness before your surgery, you will probably continue to feel that discomfort. Discomfort that comes and goes with your period is not a sign of breast cancer. If you no longer menstruate, pick a day, such as the first day of the month, to do BSE.

A breast examination has two parts, the visual exam and the palpation (touch) exam. During the visual examination, you will look at yourself in a mirror. During the palpation exam, you will use your hands to examine yourself. If you find any changes, show them to your doctors.

THE VISUAL EXAMINATION

Stand in front of a mirror. Hold your hands (palms side down) in front of you. Compare your unaffected hand to your affected hand. Notice if you have any swelling in your affected hand. Then, with your arms at your side, look in the mirror and compare the size of your arms. Do you notice any swelling? If so, you may be developing lymphedema and should make an appointment to begin treatment.

Next, with arms at your side, stand and examine your breasts and whole chest area from your collarbone to your lower bra line, and from the middle of your chest to your underarm area.

Raise your hands above your head. Slowly, turn from side to side, so that you can examine from the middle of your chest to your underarm area.

Radiation therapy may cause changes in the appearance of your breast. It is important to discuss these changes with your radiation therapist to assure yourself that the changes are normal and no cause for concern. Your treated breast may:

◆ Appear darker in color

◆ Have enlarged pores

◆ Appear more uplifted than the other breast

◆ Appear darker around the nipple and areola

If you notice any of the following changes, show them to your doctor:

◆ Persistent rash, redness, or discoloration on your breast, chest, and/or scar

◆ Persistent itchy rash on your nipple or areola

◆ Spontaneous and persistent nipple discharge

◆ A change in the shape of your breast, such as a dimple

◆ A lump in your breast, chest, and/or scar

THE PALPATION EXAMINATION

*D*uring the palpation examination, you will use your hands to examine yourself.

Lie on your back and use the hand opposite your breast to examine yourself. For example, if you are examining your right side, use your left hand.

If your breast size is a B-cup or larger, the following position will spread your breast tissue evenly over your chest. Turn on your side with your knees bent, as if you were going to sleep on your side; then turn your upper body away from your bent knees, so that your chest faces the ceiling.

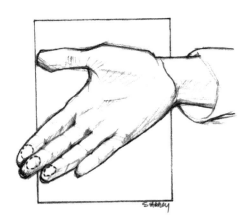

Hold your hand flat and use the fleshy pads of your middle three fingers, rather than the tips.

At each spot you examine, move the pads of your fingers in three small circles — about the size of a dime. Use three levels of pressure — light, medium, and deep. When pressing deeply, try to feel your ribs. Your ribs will feel like a washboard.

A good examination pattern is the "vertical strip method." Always start in your armpit and examine down toward your bra line.

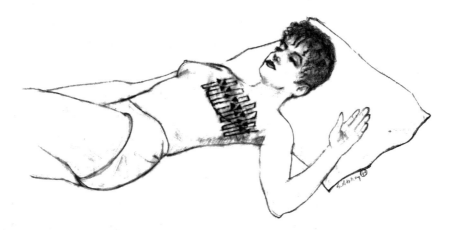

When you examine the side of your lumpectomy, pay particular attention to your scar. If you notice a hard lump, a thickening, or any change, show it to your doctor. Radiation therapy may cause changes in the way the treated breast feels on examination. If you notice any of these changes talk to your radiation oncologist to assure yourself that these changes are normal and no cause for concern. The treated breast may feel as follows:

◆ Denser and firmer.

◆ The skin on the nipple and areola may feel thicker.

◆ When exerting pressure on the breast, it may feel smoother and less lumpy to the touch.

◆ More tender to touch.

INDIVIDUAL INSTRUCTION IN BSE

*M*ost women benefit from individual instruction in BSE. Individual instruction will teach you how to hold your hand, how deeply to press, how to know what your ribs feel like, and how to sort out a lump from the normal lumpy feeling of your breast.

Ask your doctor or nurse to spend some time with you reviewing BSE. You can also check with your doctors or hospital to see whether there is a nurse who can teach you BSE.

The Mammatech Corporation has developed an effective, step-by-step home teaching program that includes a lifelike breast model and a 45-minute videotape. The breast model helps you distinguish a lump from the normal lumpy feeling of the breast; the tape reviews the visual and touch examination. Turn to the *Resource Guide* under "Breast Self-Examination" for information on obtaining the videotape.

Remember, you are the best judge of your own body — don't ever feel embarrassed to bring a change or concern to the attention of your nurse or doctor.

You may find that when examining yourself, you become anxious about finding a new lump, or even sad, because it brings up your recent experience with breast cancer. You may also feel uncertain about what you are looking or feeling for. These reactions are normal and understandable. Talking with your doctor, your social worker, or other breast cancer survivors about these feelings can help you deal with them. Asking for individual instruction in BSE can help you feel more confident about your skills.

Also, it can be helpful to think about BSE in a new light. Think of BSE as a way to get familiar with your new body, not as a way to "find cancer." Make BSE a positive affirmation of your health. After you examine yourself, you could say to yourself, "My breasts look healthy; my breasts feel healthy; my breasts are healthy."

In Conclusion

Each day, it may be helpful for you to remind yourself that you are not alone. Over 180,000 women in this country are diagnosed with breast cancer every year. These women have found in themselves and through others the strength and resources to recover and heal. Think of this community of survivors; tell yourself that you are not alone; affirm each day your belief that you, too, will recover and heal.

We hope that this guide has contributed to your recovery and healing.

Appendices

Glossary

areola: The darker part of the breast surrounding the nipple.

axilla: The armpit area that contains lymph nodes, lymph and blood vessels, fat, and muscle.

axillary lymph nodes: The lymph nodes that are located in the armpit region. Breast cancer cells can travel to the lymph nodes. So, some of these lymph nodes are removed to test them for the presence of cancer cells.

axillary lymph node dissection: The surgical removal of most of the lymph nodes found in the armpit region.

axillary lymph nodes sampling: The surgical removal of some of the lymph nodes found in the armpit region.

breast reconstruction: The surgical creation of the breast contour, nipple, and areola. Performed by a plastic surgeon.

breast self-examination (BSE): The examination of the breast, chest, and lymph nodes by a woman herself.

chemotherapy: Cancer treatment using cytotoxic (cell killing) drugs. Chemotherapy is administered when there is the risk that cancer cells have spread outside of the breast.

clinical breast examination: An examination of the breast, chest, and lymph nodes performed by a health care provider. The examination consists of a visual and a touch (palpation) examination.

ducts: The channels in the breast that carry milk out to the nipple.

estrogen: A female hormone. *See hormone assay test.*

hormone assay test: The tumor is tested to see whether the cells are receptive to estrogen and progesterone. This procedure is helpful in determining whether the cancer cells are slow or fast-growing. It is also helpful when you and your doctors are considering the use of tamoxifen (Novadex).

immune system: The body's system to promote healing and to kill viruses, bacteria, and cancer cells.

inspection: To examine visually.

invasive or infiltrating breast cancer: Breast cancer that has broken out of the milk ducts and/or lobules and invaded the surrounding breast tissue. An invasive or infiltrating cancer does not imply that the cancer is fast-growing or has spread outside of the breast.

lobules: The part of the breast that produces milk.

lumpectomy: A surgical procedure that removes the cancer and a rim of healthy tissue around the tumor. This breast conservation procedure is usually followed by five to seven weeks of radiation therapy to the breast and chest.

lymphedema: The chronic swelling of the hand and/or arm. This condition is a possible lifelong complication from removing and/or radiating the lymph nodes under the arm on the side of the lumpectomy. Lymphedema can and should be treated. Left untreated, your hand or arm can continue to get larger.

lymph nodes: Small bean-shaped glands found throughout the body that help eliminate bacteria, viruses, and cancer cells.

mastectomy: The surgical removal of the breast. A modified radical mastectomy removes the breast and some of the lymph nodes under the arm. A simple mastectomy removes the breast.

metastasis: The spread of breast cancer cells to another organ, such as the lungs, liver, brain, or bone.

oncology: The study of cancer.

oncology nurse: A nurse who specializes in the care and recovery of persons with cancer. She or he is a good resource for information on support groups, books, and videos.

oncologist: A doctor who specializes in the treatment of cancer, such as a "radiation oncologist," who specializes in the treatment of cancer with radiation therapy; a "medical oncologist," who specializes in the treatment of cancer with medication; or a "surgical oncologist," who specializes in the treatment of cancer with surgery.

pathologist: A doctor who specializes in examining tissue under a microscope and diagnosing disease.

palpation: Examination by touch.

pectoralis major and minor: The major muscles that lie under the breast and over the rib cage.

plastic surgeon: A doctor who specializes in surgically creating a breast contour, nipple, and areola.

progesterone: A female hormone. *See* hormone assay tests.

tamoxifen (Novadex): Medication for breast cancer that reduces the rate of recurrence.

Questions to Ask Your Doctors

QUESTIONS BEFORE SURGERY

◆ What kind of procedure are you recommending?

◆ How much tissue will be removed?

◆ Where will the incision be located and how large will it be?

◆ What will my breast look like after the lumpectomy?

◆ What are the risks and side effects of a lumpectomy?

◆ What type of anesthesia will I have? Local? General?

◆ How long will I be in the hospital? Same day discharge? Overnight?

AXILLARY NODE SURGERY QUESTIONS

◆ Are the lymph nodes in my armpit going to be removed?

◆ About how many lymph nodes will be removed?

◆ Where will the incision be located and how large will it be?

◆ What will my underarm area look like after the axillary node sampling/dissection?

◆ What are the risks and side effects of an axillary node sampling?

◆ How long will I be in the hospital? Same day discharge? Overnight?

Notes

QUESTIONS REGARDING RADIATION TREATMENT

◆ How long will the daily treatments last?

◆ How long will I be in the radiation therapy department?

◆ How many weeks will the treatment take?

◆ What are the risks and benefits?

◆ What are the common short-term side effects?

◆ What are the common long-term side effects?

◆ What can be done to reduce the side effects?

◆ How often will I need to see you after treatment ends?

QUESTIONS REGARDING TAMOXIFEN

◆ What are the risks and benefits of taking tamoxifen?

◆ What are some of the possible side effects of tamoxifen?

◆ How long do I need to take it?

◆ How often do I need to have a pap smear and pelvic examination?

◆ Do I need any other tests on a regular basis if I take tamoxifen?

Notes

QUESTIONS REGARDING CHEMOTHERAPY

◆ What medications do you suggest?

◆ How effective are these drugs in cases similar to mine?

◆ What are the risks and benefits?

◆ How long will I be on chemotherapy?

◆ How often do I come in for treatments?

◆ When will I receive chemotherapy, before or after radiation therapy?

◆ What are the common side effects of chemotherapy?

◆ What can be done to reduce the side effects?

◆ Will I be able to work while on chemotherapy?

◆ How often will I need to see you after treatment ends?

QUESTIONS AFTER YOUR TREATMENT IS COMPLETED

◆ How often do I need to return for examinations?

◆ How often do I need to have a mammogram?

◆ What other kinds of tests do I need to have, and how often do they need to be done?

Notes

Drain Care Chart

Record the date and the amount of drainage in the appropriate column.

DATE	MORNING	EVENING	TOTAL

Resource Guide

KEY TO RESOURCE GUIDE

*T*he resources included in this guide are selective. They were chosen because they are considered to be the best available.

1. APPEARANCE

Books

Beauty & Cancer. Dane Doan Noyes and Peggy Mellody, R.N. Taylor Pub., Dallas, Texas, 1992, 163 pages. The authors have customized makeup, wardrobe, and other beauty concerns to the specific needs of a woman undergoing chemotherapy, radiation therapy, and/or surgery. The guide covers the wearing of scarves, wigs, makeup, and clothing. Contact:

> Taylor Publishing
> 1550 South Mockingbird Lane
> Dallas, Texas 75235
> 1-800-275-8188

Breast Forms

Coloplast/Amoena manufactures a partial breast form that can be used after a lumpectomy. The partial breast form enlarges the size of the breast(s). It slips into a bra and is made of silicone for a lifelike feel. For the nearest dealer, contact:

> Coloplast, Inc.
> 1955 West Oak Circle
> Marietta, Georgia 30062
> 1-800-741-0078

Programs

Look Good. Feel Better. A free workshop for women undergoing treatment for cancer. The workshop covers using turbans, scarves, wigs, and makeup. Sponsored by the Cosmetic, Toiletry and Fragrance Association Foundation in partnership with the American Cancer Society and the National Cosmetology Association. Contact:

> 1-800-395-LOOK (1-800-395-5665)

2. Breast Self-Examination

Programs

Mammatech Corporation has developed an effective step-by-step home program to teach breast self-examination. It includes a lifelike breast model and a 45-minute videotape. The breast model helps women distinguish a lump from the normal lumpy feeling of the breast. Contact:

> Mammatech Corporation
> 930 Northwest 8th Avenue
> Gainesville, Florida 32601
> 1-800-626-2273

American Cancer Society (ACS). ACS public education programs teach breast self-examination. For services in your area call:

> 1-800-ACS-2345 (1-800-227-2345)

3. EMOTIONAL RECOVERY

Audiotapes

Voices in the Night: The Early Breast Cancer Program. Joy S. McDiarmid and Dawn M. Holman, producers. A helpful and inspiring six-tape program (five cassettes/five hours) for the patient-listener and one cassette (90 minutes) for the partner/spouse. Interwoven with conversations from long-time survivors and women recently diagnosed with breast cancer is commentary from well-known breast cancer specialists.

> Voices in the Night, Inc.
> P.O. Box 24059, 1853 Grant Avenue
> Winnipeg, M.B. R3N 2B1, Canada
> 1 800-268-0009

Books

No Less a Woman: Ten Women Shatter the Myths About Breast Cancer. Deborah H. Kahane, M.S.W. Prentice-Hall Press, 1990, 279 pages. Ten women discuss their personal stories and strategies for coping. Positive and inspiring. Written by a psychotherapist who is a breast cancer survivor. In bookstores.

Spinning Straw into Gold: Your Emotional Recovery from Breast Cancer. Ronnie Kaye, M.F.C.C. Fireside/Simon & Schuster, Inc., 1991, Paperback. 224 pages. Written by a psychotherapist who is a breast cancer survivor. In bookstores.

Invisible Scars. Mimi Greenberg, Ph.D. St. Martin's Press, New York, 1988, 204 pages. A down-to-earth, helpful, practical guide to coping with the emotional impact of breast cancer. Written by a psychotherapist who is a breast cancer survivor. In bookstores.

Pamphlet

For Single Woman with Breast Cancer. Y-Me. 1994, 40 pages. A free and helpful pamphlet that covers a wide range of issues such as dating, intimacy, sexuality, pregnancy, health insurance coverage, and employment. Contact:

> Y-Me
> 212 W. Van Buren Street
> Chicago, Illinois 60607
> 1-800-221-2141

Programs

The *YWCA Encore Program.* This program offers local support groups and exercises classes after breast surgery. Contact:

> YWCA Encore Program
> YWCA National Headquarters
> 726 Broadway
> New York, New York 10003
> 1-212-614-2700

Reach for Recovery Program. This free program is run by local chapters of the American Cancer Society (ACS). Provides one-to-one emotional support and information. Trained volunteers are breast cancer survivors. They can visit you at home or in the hospital. For services in your area call:

> 1-800-ACS-2345 (1-800-227-2345)

4. EXERCISE

Videos

Beginning Ballet for the Post-Lumpectomy Woman. Pattie Bryson, breast cancer survivor, nurse, and ballet instructor, demonstrates step-by-step instruction that encourages flexibility and upper-body strengthening. 50 min. Order from:

> First Position Production
> Star Route Box 472
> Sausalito California 94965
> 1-415-381-3403

Get Up and Go. After Breast Surgery. Exercise program that includes warm-up, wall and pole exercises, stretching and toning, and meditation. Order by mail or phone:

> Health Tapes, Inc.
> 13320 North End Avenue
> Oak Park, Michigan 48237
> 1-810-548-2500

Programs

YWCA Encore Program. Water and floor exercises specially developed for women who have had breast cancer surgery. A woman can join the group as early as three weeks after surgery. Call your local YWCA or contact the national office:

> YWCA Encore Program
> YWCA National Headquarters
> 726 Broadway
> New York, New York 10003
> 1-212-614-2700

5. HEALTH INSURANCE

Books

An Almanac of Practical Resources for Cancer Survivors, Charting the Journey. National Coalition for Cancer Survivorship (NCCS). Consumers Union, 1990, 225 pages. A comprehensive collection of resources. Includes information and strategies to help with health insurance concerns. Order from:

> NCCS
> 1010 Wayne Avenue, 7th Floor
> Silver Spring, Maryland 20910
> 1-301-650-8868

6. LYMPHEDEMA

Books and Pamphlets

Recovery in Motion. Linda T. Miller, P.T. 1992, 13 pages. An exercise program to assist in the management of upper extremity lymphedema. To order, contact:

> Linda T. Miller, P.T.
> Breast Cancer Physical Therapy Center, Ltd.
> 1905 Spruce Street
> Philadelphia, Pennsylvania 19103
> 1-215-772-0160

Organization

The *National Lymphedema Network* (NLN). The NLN provides education regarding the prevention and treatment of lymphedema. Hotline offers support, information, and referrals for treatment of lymphedema. Quarterly newsletter. Contact:

> National Lymphedema Network
> 2211 Post Street, Suite 404
> San Francisco, California 94115
> 1-800-541-3259

7. MENOPAUSE

Books

Dr. Susan Lark's Menopause Self-Help Book. Susan M. Lark. M.D. Celestial Books, 1990, 239 pages. Provides a workbook for evaluating menopausal symptoms and a natural approach for relieving symptoms. Recipes. In bookstores. Also call:

> LifeCycles
> 1-800-862-9876

Natural Menopause. Susan Perry and Katherine O'Hanlan, M.D. Addison-Wesley Publishing Co., 1992, 300 pages. A user-friendly book that explains the physical and emotional changes that menopause can bring. Explores a lifestyle that encourages optimum health and symptom relief. In bookstores.

8. NUTRITION

Books and Pamphlets

Eating Hints: Recipes and Tips for Better Nutrition During Cancer Treatment. 1990, 95 pages. This free cookbook-style booklet includes recipes and suggestions for maintaining optimum yet realistic nutrition during treatment. Originally produced by the Yale-New Haven Medical Center and reprinted by the National Cancer Institute. Contact:

> Cancer Information Service
> 1-800-422-6237

9. ORGANIZATIONS

American Cancer Society (ACS). A national non-profit organization with local chapters that provides education and patient service programs. "Reach for Recovery" is a program that provides one-to-one emotional support and information by trained volunteers who are breast cancer survivors. "Look Good. Feel Better." is a free workshop for woman undergoing treatment for cancer. The workshop covers using turbans, scarves, wigs, and makeup. For services in your area call:

> 1-800-ACS-2345 (1-800-227-2345)

Breast Cancer Action. This is an activist and advocacy organization of breast cancer survivors and their supporters whose purpose is to increase the awareness of breast cancer among those in government, the scientific community, private industry, and the media. They have an excellent bi-monthly newsletter. Contact:

> Breast Cancer Action
> 55 New Montgomery St., Suite 624
> San Francisco, California 94105
> 1-415-243-9301

National Alliance of Breast Cancer Organizations (NABCO). Provides information on breast cancer as well as information on regional organizations that offer support to breast cancer survivors. Quarterly newsletter. Contact:

> NABCO
> 9 East 37th Street, 10th Floor
> New York, New York 10016
> 1-212-719-0154

Susan G. Komen Breast Cancer Foundation. A national organization that supports breast cancer research, education, screening, and treatment. Trained volunteers answer a helpline to provide emotional support, information, and support group referrals. Contact:

1-800-IM-AWARE (1-800-462-9273)

The *Cancer Information Service* (CIS) of the National Cancer Institute (NCI). The NCI is part of the National Institute of Health and is the federal government's principal agency for cancer research and control. The CIS offers free written material and information about treatment, support services, medical facilities, second opinion centers, and clinical trials. Trained information specialists answer cancer-related questions. Call:

1-800-4-CANCER (1-800-422-6237)

The *National Coalition for Cancer Survivorship* (NCCS). The NCCS is a national coalition of individuals, organizations, and institutions dedicated to survivorship and support of people with cancer and their families. This organization helps locate support groups and resources, serves as an advocate for the rights of cancer survivors, and promotes the study of survivorship. Quarterly newsletter. Contact:

NCCS
1010 Wayne Avenue, 7th Floor
Silver Spring, Maryland 20910
1-301-650-8868

Y-Me National Breast Organization for Cancer Information and Support. Y-Me is a non-profit organization providing information, peer support, and referral. It also offers information on treatment options, workshops, and supports groups. Y-Me has chapters throughout the country that offer local support group meetings. Callers can talk with trained volunteers who are breast cancer survivors. Contact:

Y-Me
212 W. Van Buren Street
Chicago, Illinois 60607
1-800-221-2141

10. RELAXATION

Catalogue

Living Arts. A beautifully designed mail-order catalogue that contains books, videos, and audiotapes on yoga, mediation, and relaxation.

Living Arts
P.O. Box 2939
Venice, California 90291-2939
1-800-254-8464

11. RESOURCES FOR PARTNERS

Books and Pamphlets

Cancer in Two Voices. Sandra Butler and Barbara Rosenbaum. Spinster Book Co., San Francisco, 1991, 183 pages. Using essays, journal entries, and letters, two women share the experience of living with breast cancer and of being the partner who survives. The authors transform the sorrow of cancer into a celebration of life. In bookstores.

When the Woman You Love Has Breast Cancer. Larry T. Eiler. Queen Bee Publishing Co., 1994, 36 pages. A personal account. A husband talks frankly about such issues as coping with emotions and getting support, helping his children cope, sexuality, and suggestions for husbands. Contact:

> Queen Bee Publishing Co.
> 900 Victor's Way, Suite 180
> Ann Arbor, Michigan 48108
> 1-313-761-3399

When the Woman You Love Has Breast Cancer. Y-Me. 1994, 16 pages. A free pamphlet written for men. It provides helpful suggestions to improve communication, physical closeness, and sexual intimacy. Contact:

> Y-Me
> 212 W. Van Buren Street
> Chicago, Illinois 60607
> 1-800-221-2141

Videos

The Male Perspective: Husbands Talk About Their Wives and Breast Cancer. Four husbands talk frankly about such issues as the diagnosis and how they reacted, coping with emotions and getting support, helping their children cope, physical issues, sexuality, and suggestions for husbands. To order, send a check for $41.00 to:

> Kathy LaTour
> The Breast Cancer Companion Tapes
> P.O. Box 141182
> Dallas, Texas 75214

Cancer in Two Voices. An inspiring 43-minute film on the relationship between two women — one with terminal breast cancer — as they live a life of humor and candor the three years before the partner's death. Their courage and creativity are life-affirming. To order, call:

> Sandbar Production
> 1-707-944-0706

12. Sexual Intimacy

Books and Pamphlets

Sexuality and Cancer: For the Woman Who Has Cancer, and Her Partner. 1988, 40 pages. This free booklet gives clear, honest information about cancer and sexuality. American Cancer Society publication. Call:

> 1-800-ACS-2345 (1-800-227-2345)

Up Front: Sex and the Post-Mastectomy Woman. Linda Dackman. Penguin paperback, 1991, 128 pages. Honest, intimate, and funny account by a single woman who is a breast cancer survivor in her 30s. In bookstores.

Organizations

American Association of Sex Educators, Counselors, and Therapists (AASECT). A professional organization of trained sex educators, counselors, and therapists. For a list of qualified therapists in your state, send a $2.00 check or money order and a self-addressed stamped envelope to:

> AASECT
> 435 North Michigan Avenue, Suite 1717
> Chicago, Illinois 60611-4067
> 1-312-644-0828

Products

Astroglide. A non-prescription, water-based vaginal lubricant. It is free of scents or flavors. If you would like more information, contact:

> Bio Film, Inc.
> 3121 Scott Street
> Vista, California 92083
> 1-800-325-5695

Probe. A non-prescription, water-based vaginal lubricant. It is tasteless, odorless, exceptionally slippery, and composed primarily of water. If you would like more information, contact:

> Davryan Laboratories, Inc.
> 2623 S.W. Park Place
> Portland, Oregon 97201
> 1-800-637-7623

Replense. A non-prescription vaginal lotion that replenishes vaginal moisture. It is greaseless, non-staining, fragrance free, non-irritating, and contains no estrogen. If you would like more information, contact:

> Warner-Lambert Co.
> Parke-Davis
> Morris Plains, New Jersey 07950
> 1-800-524-2624

13. TREATMENT

Books

Choices in Healing: Integrating the Best of Conventional and Complementary Approaches to Cancer. Michael Lerner, Ph.D. Cambridge: MIT Press, 1994, 340 pages. This comprehensive book provides accurate and realistic information about conventional and complementary therapies. Complementary therapies is the main focus, with major sections on spirituality, pharmacology, and nutrition. In bookstores. Order through:

> Commonweal
> P.O. Box 316
> Bolinas, California 94924
> 1-415-868-2642

Coping with Chemotherapy. Nancy Bruning. Ballantine Books, New York, 1992, 327 pages. A comprehensive overview of the medical, physical, and emotional aspects of chemotherapy written by a breast cancer survivor who had chemotherapy. Contains a list of standard drugs and their side effects, and a glossary of terms. In bookstores.

The Chemotherapy Survival Guide. Judith McKay, R.N., and Nancee Hirano, R.N., M.S.N. New Harbinger Publications, 1993, 187 pages. A reader-friendly, concise guide that contains information that optimizes health and reduces side effects while on chemotherapy. A very good chapter on relaxation and stress reduction. In bookstores.

Dr. Susan Love's Breast Book. Susan M. Love, M.D. and Karen Lindsey. Addison-Wesley, 1990, 455 pages. Written by a surgeon. This popular book has become the "bible" for the newly diagnosed women. It provides an easy-to-understand presentation of all aspects of breast cancer from diagnosis to recovery. In bookstores.

Index

Authors

Rosalind D. Benedet, N.P., M.S.N., has also written *Healing — A Woman's Guide To Recovery After Mastectomy.* She is the Coordinator of the Breast Cancer Recovery Program at the Breast Health Center of California Pacific Medical Center in San Francisco, California. She received her nursing degree and a Master's in Nursing Science at the M.G.H. Institute of Health Professions in Boston, Massachusetts. Rosalind is a certified nurse practitioner in women's health. She is a native of San Francisco.

Mark C. Rounsaville, M.D., is a board-certified radiation oncologist in practice at California Pacific Medical Center, San Francisco. He is an advocate of patient self-responsibility through education. He has long supported the importance of quality of life issues in health care.

Editor

Edith (Edie) L. Folb, Ph.D., is a professor of Speech and Communication Studies at San Francisco State University. She has taught a variety of courses during her 17 years at SFSU, including intercultural communication, interpersonal communication, oral literature, and women's communicative behavior. She has published extensively on topics ranging from women's language and culture to African American language use to multicultural education. Before coming to SFSU, she taught at UCLA, UCSD, UC Irvine, and at the Women's Building in Los Angeles. She has long been an advocate of women's rights in education and health care.

Illustrator

Shannon K. Abbey is an illustrator and painter in San Francisco. She teaches drawing at the Academy of Art College and is a member of the San Francisco Society of Illustrators.

Shannon can be reached weekdays at her Potrero Hill studio, (415) 252-0199.

Production Manager

M.J. Coleman, wife, mother, and professional, has spent her working career in the creative field, serving as Vice President, Creative Services for Bank of America; heading her own design company, M.J. Coleman Design; and currently representing San Francisco-based Heiney & Craig, Inc., one of the largest annual report and collateral design firms in California.

"After having a bilateral mastectomy and reconstructive surgery in 1993, I was disappointed with the limited amount of information available for women like me. I wished there had been a book that answered so many of the questions I had before and after my surgery. When asked to assist with *Healing — A Woman's Guide to Recovery After Mastectomy*, I didn't hesitate because I knew there were others like me looking for answers."

Financial Contribution

Dr. Richard Cohen Cancer Fund of the California Pacific Medical Center in San Francisco, California, provided a generous grant that made the printing of this book possible.

Sharron Long was diagnosed with breast cancer the same year her sister Judy Hill died of the disease. Her association with the author is the result of her desire to make a contribution to the breast cancer community in her sister's name; hence, the dedication of this book. It is her hope that this will be a "working" memorial to her sister in that it will help breast cancer patients everywhere deal with their diagnosis and begin their healing process.

Quantity	Price	Shipping	Tax
1	$12.00	$1.50	$1.02
10	$70.00	$6.00	$5.95
70	$438.00	$21.00	$37.23

Please send me:

_____copy(ies) *Healing:* **A Woman's Guide To Recovery After Mastectomy** $_____

_____copy(ies) *Healing:* **A Woman's Guide To Lumpectomy and Radiation Therapy** $_____

Shipping $_____

Sales Tax (CA Residents Only) $_____

TOTAL $_____

☐ Send me_____brochures

DATE _____

NAME _____

COMPANY NAME _____

ADDRESS_____

_____

PHONE _____

ALL ORDERS MUST BE PREPAID

Make check payable to:
Benedet Publishing
220 Montgomery Street
Penthouse No. 2
San Francisco, CA 94104
(415) 281-3380